Handbook of

MRI
SCANNING

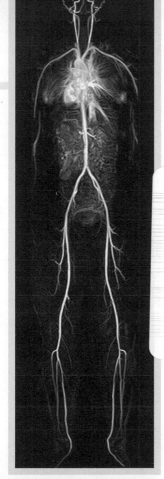

Geraldine Burghart, MA, RT(R)(MR)(M)
Associate Professor
Radiologic Technology Program
Department of Nursing and Allied Health Sciences
City University of New York, BCC
Bronx, New York

Carol Ann Finn, RT(R)(MR)
Manager, MRI Department
New York—Presbyterian Hospital,
Columbia Campus, New York,
New York

ELSEVIER
MOSBY

3251 Riverport Lane
St. Louis, Missouri 63043

HANDBOOK OF MRI SCANNING
ISBN: 978-0-323-06818-5

Notices

Knowledge and best practice in this field are constantly changing. As new research and experience broaden our understanding, changes in research methods, professional practices, or medical treatment may become necessary.

Practitioners and researchers must always rely on their own experience and knowledge in evaluating and using any information, methods, compounds, or experiments described herein. In using such information or methods they should be mindful of their own safety and the safety of others, including parties for whom they have a professional responsibility.

With respect to any drug or pharmaceutical products identified, readers are advised to check the most current information provided (i) on procedures featured or (ii) by the manufacturer of each product to be administered, to verify the recommended dose or formula, the method and duration of administration, and contraindications. It is the responsibility of practitioners, relying on their own experience and knowledge of their patients, to make diagnoses, to determine dosages and the best treatment for each individual patient, and to take all appropriate safety precautions.

To the fullest extent of the law, neither the Publisher nor the Authors, contributors, or editors, assume any liability for any injury and/or damage to persons or property as a matter of products liability, negligence or otherwise, or from any use or operation of any methods, products, instructions, or ideas contained in the material herein.

ISBN: 978-0-323-06818-5

Acquisitions Editor: Jeanne Olson
Developmental Editor: Luke Held
Publishing Services Manager: Julie Eddy
Senior Project Manager: Andrea Campbell
Design Direction: Maggie Reid

Printed in India
Last digit is the print number: 13

Dedication

We would like to thank our families for their continued support and encouragement throughout this lengthy process

and

We acknowledge our colleagues at New York Presbyterian Hospital for their dedication to this ever-evolving segment of Diagnostic Imaging.

Foreword

Those of us witnessing the development of magnetic resonance imaging (MRI) technology in the early years could hardly envision the extent to which routine MRI and MR angiography (MRA) is performed on every organ system of the body today. Those primitive time-consuming early simple scans involving primarily T1- and T2-weighted imaging have evolved into fast, complex examinations involving many more contrast mechanisms, often with very precise positioning of the imaging plane relative to the anatomic structures. This has resulted from a spectacular explosion of refinements to MR capability involving improvements in magnets, shimming, gradient coils, rf coils, pulse sequences, data transmission, image reconstruction algorithms, user interfaces, and contrast agents. Along with these advances have been some much needed automation and simplifications to the operation of MR scanners. However, on the whole, the MR scanners are fantastically more complicated, demanding technologists and radiologists of the highest caliber for successful implementation of the latest techniques.

In spite of the complexity of MRI today, the demand for MRI remains insatiable. In radiology departments around the world,

MRI scanners are humming with patients late at night long after computed tomography, ultrasound, and nuclear medicine have closed down for the evening. Heightened concern over exposure to ionizing radiation, exquisite soft tissue detail, and availability of extraordinarily safe contrast agents have all contributed to the appeal of MRI. Claustrophobia, a downside to the top-of-the-line high-field magnets, is being gradually eliminated with shorter, larger-bore magnet architectures. This growing demand and complexity of MRI and its expansion into all parts of the body are making it imperative that we find a way to rapidly and effectively train technologists and radiologists in applying this technology to best advantage.

This book presents an outstanding, comprehensive introduction to MRI throughout the body in a practical, realistic approach that avoids confusing physics and equations. Starting out with safety, it then systematically steps through the body by MR anatomic regions, treating each in a standardized fashion so that the information is easily assimilated. The basic approaches to each body part are supplemented with myriad insights, reflecting the genius and wealth of experience of the authors,

Carol Finn and Geri Burghart. Carol Finn has been an MRI specialist for more than 20 years, with experience in academic universities, private practice, and imaging centers, as well as extensive experience teaching MRI and training technologists and radiologists. Geri Burghart is an Associate Professor and has also been an educator in radiologic technology for more than 20 years. Accordingly, this book represents a must-read for all beginning MRI technologists and will be a great resource for experienced technologists and MR radiologists.

Martin R. Prince, MD, PhD, FACR
Professor of Radiology Weill Cornell Medical Center and
Columbia College of Physicians and Surgeons,
New York City, September 20, 2010

The fMRI Team

Performing clinical fMRI studies is a complex process that requires close cooperation and team work between the physician and the technologist. The physician is responsible for planning and interpretation of these studies but cannot perform the fMRI acquisition without the help of the technologist. In addition, at our institution, after the physician sets the protocol and explains the fMRI process to the patient, it is the technologist who assumes the responsibility for monitoring the performance of the fMRI tasks. We have progressively given this responsibility to our technologists as they have acquired more knowledge and mastered each stage of the process. This has proven to be a very workable relationship and because our technologists have taken "ownership" of the process, they routinely take the initiative to adapt paradigms and find creative ways to compensate for the many limitations we encounter in our challenging neurological ICU patient population. This integral role of the technologist in the process of performing fMRI studies emphasizes the need for technologists to have an in-depth understanding of the scientific underpinnings of fMRI. This also applies to the acquisition of other specialized "functional" MRI studies, including diffusion, diffusion tensor, perfusion and spectroscopy. The fMRI section in Chapter 1 provides an overview of these advanced MRI techniques to help technologists get started developing the knowledge base they will need to participate as a key member of the imaging team doing advanced MRI studies.

Robert L. DeLaPaz, MD
Director of Neuroradiology
CIO & Director of PACS
Department of Radiology
New York Presbyterian Hospital, Columbia Medical Center
New York City, September 25, 2010

Reviewers

Lynda Donathan, MS, RT(R)(M)(CT)(MR)
Assistant Professor of Imaging Sciences
Morehead State University
Morehead, Kentucky

Cheryl O. DuBose, MSRS, RT(R)(MR)(CT)(QM)
MRI Program Chair
Arkansas State University
Jonesboro, Arkansas

Michael Teters, MS, DABR
Assistant Professor
UMDNJ-SHRP
Scotch Plains, New Jersey

Patricia L. Tyhurst, BAEd, CPC, CPCH
Department Chair
University of Montana
Helena, Montana

Acknowledgments

In addition to the reviewers listed separately, the authors would like to thank the following individuals for their contributions:

Robert DeLaPaz, MD
Professor of Radiology
Director of Neuroradiology,
NYP Columbia Medical Center
Foreword "MD-Technologist interaction" and fMRI section images and context.

Martin R. Prince, MD, PhD, FACR
Professor of Radiology at Cornell & Columbia Universities
Foreword and review of the contrast section

Cindy R, Comeau, BS, RT(N)(MR)
Advanced Cardiovascular Imaging, NY, NY
Provided images for the cardiac section

Cover image courtesy of Mitsue Miyazaki from Toshiba Medical Systems Corp.

Caption: The entire arterial vasculature is depicted with exquisite clarity using noncontrast angiography techniques. The fresh blood imaging (FBI) technique was used to depict the pulmonary system, subclavian arteries, and runoff vessels, from the abdominal aorta to the pedal arteries. The time-spatial labeling inversion pulse (Time-SLIP) technique was used to depict the carotid arteries through the Circle of Willis.

Contents

CONTENTS

Preface

As both technologists and educators, we strongly believe there is a need for a comprehensive reference for MR scanning. This includes not only the accurate and consistently standardized acquisition of images, but also a place to reference standard and advanced protocols for imaging the vast range of medical conditions and body habitus presented.

We feel this book is both basic and broad enough to meet the needs of students and experienced technologists. It is intended to provide not only a baseline for MR image acquisition but also a standard of quality that should be consistently duplicated to provide the health care team with quality diagnostic images.

In our tables we have suggested scan protocols with technical parameters for both 1.5T and the more advanced 3T magnets. In addition we have provided blank tables to modify your site protocols to accommodate the capabilities of your specific equipment. We suggest you enter all data on your site tables in pencil to modify as protocols and software change.

Of utmost importance, regardless of the field strength of your specific equipment, is MR safety. MR safety guidelines, as set forth by your facility and the MR technologist, is the first line of defense against MR related accidents. Included in this text is an overview of MR safety including issues related to administration of contrast agents .We urge all MR personnel to adhere to all safety protocols to avoid accidents that can injure patients, staff and equipment.

ORGANIZATION AND CONTENT

- A safety section, including MR suite configuration, patient screening and personnel classifications, provides a solid foundation for secure operating parameters within the highly volatile MR environment.
- A section on Gadolinium Based Contrast Agents (GBCAs) provides background on safety considerations as outlined by the ACR, pharmaceutical vendors, including appropriate dosing and off label use.
- Each section is logically divided into protocols for acquisition in the axial, coronal and sagittal planes, with suggestions for scan parameters and sequences for both 1.5T and 3T.
- Tables suggesting protocols and sequences for both 1.5T and 3T magnets.

- Each pilot, or scan plan, is followed by a relevant midline image from the sequence and a detailed anatomical reference of the pertinent anatomy.
- The parameters for coil type, proper patient positioning, consistent and accurate slice placement and anatomical coverage are detailed for each sequence. In addition, a "Tips" section will assist with techniques designed to perfect each scan and ensure patient safety and comfort.
- The fMRI section at the end of Chapter 1 gives insight to some of the most current techniques and applications of MRI.
- The cross-vendor reference acronym chart allows replication of sequences from one vendor to another.

Each chapter has
- Scan Considerations
- Coils
- Pulse Sequences
- Options
- Scanning Tips
- Scan Planning
- Anatomic Midline Image
- Anatomic Drawing

ANCILLARIES

- The images from the book are available online on Evolve at http://evolve.elsevier.com/BurghartFinn/MRI

Patient Preparation

- The patient should be "properly identified" by name, date of birth and facility medical record number (when appropriate), which should be compared to the patient's requisition and schedule.
- Have the patient fill out a MRI questionnaire while in zone 2.
- The MRI questionnaire should be reviewed by the MRI staff, particularly nurse and the technologist who are the "gatekeepers".
- The MRI questionnaire should be discussed with the patient making sure they understand the questions.
- The patient should be screened for implanted devices, such as a pacemaker, defibrillator, neuro-stimulator, aneurysm clip, hearing aid and prosthetic devices.
- Patient should be screened for the possibility of renal disease when contrast is ordered.
- Have the patient go to the bathroom prior to coming into the MRI suite.
- All patients should undress and put on a gown or scrubs. Make sure all metal is removed.

- Many patients are anxious when having an MRI. Make sure you explain the examination to the patient. A conversation with the patient prior to scanning usually puts the patient's fears to rest.
- Explain the importance of holding still.
- Explain that the scanner makes a loud knocking sound and they should try to relax.
- Explain that you will be talking to them between scans. Give patient a call bell and instructions to use only when necessary.
- When they speak to you, make sure you listen to what they say so you can address their needs if necessary.
- Make sure ear plugs are securely fitted into the patient's ears.
- Secure the head with side sponges, and tape with gauze across the forehead.
- Secure the patient in a comfortable position, with cushions under their knees to relieve back pressure.
- Put sponges or sheets along the side of the patient to prevent their arms and torso from touching the sides of the magnet.

Safety Guidelines

MR environments can pose a wide array of potential risks for patients, health care workers, and ancillary personnel who enter the magnetic field. Strict policy and procedures should be in place and adhered to, to ensure safe operation. Areas to be considered are zoning of the MR suite, identification and education of qualified MR personnel, guidelines for screening patients and accompanying family members, administration of contrast, implant, and device screening and cryogens.

The inherent risks for accidents caused by the magnetic field continue to be similar at 1.5T and 3T. However, as the static magnetic field strength increases, the probability for movement of ferromagnetic material, metallic implants and the projectile effect become increasingly problematic. To avoid tissue heating, which is caused by the time-varying magnetic field, the FDA provides guidance on the rate of energy that may be deposited in tissue, which is termed *specific absorption rate* (SAR). In addition, the time-varying magnetic field can affect acoustic noise and induce voltage. At 3T, SAR can becomes a greater concern, particularly with fast spin echo sequences, especially as the echo train length increases. For this reason, all 3T MR vendors provide SAR monitors with their 3T magnets. These monitors should be observed while scanning.

As practitioners and educators, we strongly suggest the American College of Radiology (ACR) Guidance Document for MR Practices: 2007 (listed in the references to these Safety Guidelines) be referenced and adhered to for implementation of safety guidelines in all MRI departments. Further information for safe practice can be accessed at the Joint Commission Sentinel Event Alert on MRI Safety and at NIH.gov/mri (both links are found in the references to these Safety Guidelines). A brief overview of ACR guidelines are discussed below.

ZONING OF THE MR SUITE

The architectural plan for the MR suite should support safety and be designed with barriers to prevent harm to patients and personnel. The four-zone plan suggested by the ACR is described below. Whatever system is adopted, it should be strictly adhered to. The entrance to each zone should be clearly marked.

Zone I—All areas that are outside the MR environment and are accessible to the general public. In this area, no risk is posed to the general public.

Zone II—This is the area that bridges the contact between Zone I and the more strictly supervised areas of Zone III and IV. This is the area where patients are typically screened and history is taken.

Zone III—This is a restricted area for all who are not MR personnel. Because the magnetic field is three-dimensional and may project through walls and floors, this area should be clearly marked as potentially hazardous. The five-gauss line, which is the exclusionary zone, should be clearly delineated. Signage should be posted to ensure that all patients or staff with pacemakers or defibrillators do not enter this area.

Zone IV—This is the room in which the MR scanner is housed and is the area that poses the most potential risk. It should be clearly marked with proper signage stating: **"The Magnet is Always On,"** and that you are entering Zone IV.

MR PERSONNEL

Considering the potential dangers that can occur in the MR suite, all individuals working within this environment should be annually certified in the completion of safe practice educational training. These practitioners should be designated as MR personnel and are typically divided into two categories—level 1 and level 2 MR personnel.

Level 1 personnel—Anyone who has completed basic MR training and will be permitted in Zones I–III.

Level 2 personnel—It should be the responsibility of the MR safety officer to identify the personnel who qualify as level 2 personnel. They should possess comprehensive MR training and understand the potential for hazardous situations that may arise from a wide variety of risks associated with Zones III and IV. Level 2 personnel will primarily consist of the MR technologist and the MR nurse.

MR Technologist—As stated by the ACR, all MR technologists should be American Registry of Radiologic Technologists–certified radiologic technologists (RTs). All MR technologists should maintain current certification by the American Heart Association in basic life support at the health care provider level.

GUIDELINES FOR SCREENING PATIENTS AND NON-MR PERSONNEL

Several components of patient screening can and should take place during the scheduling process. Typically at this time, it is determined whether the patient has any contraindicated implants such as a pacemaker or internal cardiac defibrillator, or whether there is a medical condition such as renal disease or pregnancy that may need special considerations before scanning.

All patients and personnel who attempt to enter Zone III must be formally screened and documented in writing. **Only MR personnel are qualified to perform the screening process before permitting non-MR personnel into Zone III.** MR screening should be performed by at least two separate individuals, one of whom should be a level 2 MR personnel.

Screening should typically take place in Zone II, where the patients should remove all outer clothing, jewelry, and prosthetics, and change into a gown. The formal institutional screening questionnaire should include confidential information and a MR hazard checklist, which would be reviewed along with comprehensive discussion of the patient's medical history. The screening forms for patients and non- MR personnel who may accompany the patient, or enter the scan room, should essentially be the same.

Everyone entering Zone III must be physically screened for the presence of ferromagnetic materials, which, regardless of size, can become hazardous projectiles to the patient and the MR scanner. The use of a ferromagnetic detector and wand that differentiates between ferrous and nonferrous material is recommended.

Determination to scan a patient with an implanted medical device or foreign body should be made by the attending MR radiologist via plain x-ray films or computed tomography. For other implantable devices, further investigation for compatibility should be made and documented by MR personnel.

PEDIATRIC CONCERNS

Because children and teens are often unreliable sources of medical history, they should be questioned both in the presence of a parent or guardian, as well as alone to ensure that a complete history is disclosed.

Children comprise the largest group of patients for whom sedation is necessary. Although protocols will vary, strict adherence to guidelines and constant monitoring is mandatory. For infants, special attention must be paid to monitoring body temperature for both hypo- and hyperthermia.

PREGNANCY AND MR

Pregnant MR personnel are permitted to work within the confines of Zone IV during all stages of pregnancy but it is recommended that they not enter the MR room when the radiofrequency (RF) is on during the scanning process.

Because no detrimental effect of MR has been conclusively documented to the developing fetus, no special consideration is suggested for any stage of a patient's pregnancy. However, screening for pregnancy is recommended before MR, particularly when the study may require contrast. MR contrast should *not* be routinely injected during pregnancy unless risk versus benefit has been assessed.

DEVICE SCREENING

As part of Zone III safety protocol, the availability of a hand-held magnet (≥ 1000 gauss) or target scanner (wand) is recommended to clear and test equipment.

Before MR personnel enter Zone III, all metallic or partially metallic objects must be identified in writing as ferromagnetic or nonferromagnetic and safe or conditionally safe before entering this area. **Never assume MR compatibility** unless documented in writing and tested with a hand-held magnet. Every object entering Zone III must be tested and the results, including the date and the method of testing, documented in writing. In accordance with FDA labeling criteria, developed by American Society for Testing and Materials International, all metallic material must conform to the following standard.

MR Safe   MR Conditional   Not MR Safe

MR SCANNING SAFETY

Both patients and accompanying family members must be completely screened before entering Zone IV—the scan room. Both patients and those remaining in the room during the scan must wear **ear protection** to limit the noise from the magnet. Acoustic noise can reach 90 dB; the pain threshold is approximately 120 dB.

Patients with **implanted wires or leads** are at a higher risk when sequences such as echo-planar imaging in DWI, fMRI, or gradient intense sequences are used. Many factors can affect the potential for tissue heating. The strength of the magnetic field and type of sequences should be taken into consideration. Time-varying gradient fields can influence nerves, blood vessels, and muscles, which can act as conductors.

Thermal heating is of great concern during the scanning process. Heat generated by electrical voltages and currents within the magnet is sufficient to cause thermal injury or burns to the patient. RF energy transmits easily through open space from the RF transmit coil to the patient. To avoid excessive heating or damage to a patient's tissue, avoid placing any conductive material within the RF field. Only MR-compatible wires or leads may be used during the scanning process to prevent RF-induced burns. If electrically conductive materials must be used, position them to prevent "cross points" (cables that touch, loop over themselves, or come in contact with the RF coil).

During the scan process, it is imperative that the patient's tissue does not come into contact with the walls of the bore. Most vendors provide pads for this purpose. Caution should be taken that the patient's anatomy does not form conductive loops. Instruct patients not to cross their legs or clasp their hands on their torso during the scan process. These risks are of special concern at higher field and gradient strengths.

Drug patches that deliver medications may have metallic backing and are therefore at risk for delivering burns during the scan process. Consult with the patient's physician before removing the patch so the dose is not miscalculated.

In the event of a **code**, the patient should be removed from Zone IV and brought directly into Zone II. Code responders should be aware of safety implications within the MR suite.

In the event of a **quench**, when cryogens are released and sometimes form a white cloud in the scan room, it is imperative to quickly remove all patients and personnel and close the door to the scan room until the vendor engineers are present.

In the event of a **fire**, it is important to note that responding police and fire personnel must be prevented from entering the scan room with ferromagnetic objects. All MR suites should have MR-compatible, nonferrous fire extinguishers readily available.

Follow all manufacturer specifications for safe operation and maintenance of all patient monitoring equipment used during MR procedures.

All MR facilities should have a MR safety officer and committee who oversee and enforce the written MR safety policies for their institution.

There are many factors to consider for ensuring that a MR facility is properly prepared to serve patients and support MR personnel. Adaptation to the ACR Guidelines and strict adherence to the policies and procedures put into place by your institution will maximize a safe and secure environment.

References

Kanal E, Barkovich AJ, Bell C, et al: ACR Guidance Document for Safe MR Practices: 2007. Available at: http://www.acr.org/SecondaryMainMenuCategories/quality_safety/MRSafety/safe_mr07.aspx

American College of Radiology. Joint Commission Issues MRI Sentinel Event Alert. Available at: http://www.acr.org/SecondaryMainMenuCategories/quality_safety/MRSafety/JointCommissionIssuesMRISentinelEventAlert.aspx.

Mednovus: SAFESCAN Target Scanner. Available at: http://www.mednovus.com/targetscanner.html.

http://koppdevelopment.com

MRI of the Head and Neck

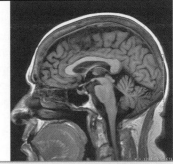

CHAPTER OUTLINE

IMPORTANT CONSIDERATIONS FOR SCAN ACQUISITION

Scan Considerations

- Refer to all vendor specific safety parameters.
- When scanning the brain, the most advantageous scan plane to cover the entire brain is the axial. Axial scans of the brain should be acquired with slices angled parallel to the genu and splenium of the corpus callosum. This enables duplication for subsequent exams of the brain.
- Be consistent when prescribing scans, i.e., put all axial slices in identical positions for each scan so the radiologist can compare one sequence with another.
- Learn to compare the hemispheres of the brain to identify pathology, paying close attention to symmetry.
- When contrast of the brain is indicated, allow adequate time before scanning. Contrast enhancement can take several minutes for maximum visualization. Today's sequences are very short and scanning too quickly after the injection will cause loss of contrast effectiveness. A radiologist may perform the T2 fluid-attenuated inversion recovery (FLAIR) or another pulse sequence after contrast to wait for the gadolinium to become more effective. Others wait a few minutes and then scan the coronal and sagittal before the axial scan. Other methods may be used as well.

Coils

- A multi-channel HD head coil or multi channel HNS (head, neck, spine) coil is recommended.
- A head or neurovascular coil can be used when necessary, i.e., some patients cannot fit in the multi-channel HD head coil.
- All multi-channel coils produce excessive signal adjacent to the coil. This can be compensated for by using vendor-specific coil intensity correction options to provide uniform signal intensity.

Pulse Sequences

- At 3T, T1 FLAIR is substituted for T1 spin echo (SE) or fast spin echo (FSE), to compensate for long T1 relaxation times at 3T.
- T1 FLAIR best differentiates gray and white mater details of the brain at 3T.
- T1 spin echo and fast spin echo, and T1 FLAIR imaging is used to best identify anatomical structure, whereas T2 and T2 FLAIR imaging provide detailed evidence of pathology.
- On T1 FLAIR and T1 sequences, cerebrospinal fluid (CSF) produces dark or hypo-intense signal. T1 FLAIR uses an inversion pulse to produce dark or hypo-intense signal.

- On T2 sequences, CSF produces bright or hyper-intense signal. T2 FLAIR uses an inversion pulse to produce dark or hypo-intense CSF signal, whereas all other abnormal fluid appears bright.
- BRAVO (BRAin VOlume imaging) are high resolution sub-millimeter isotropic T1 SPGR sequences that use an IR pulse to obtain superior gray/white matter differentiation. These can be acquired in any plane and reformatted.
- IDEAL (GE) is a fat/water separation technique (previously called 3-point Dixon technique) that can also be used to eliminate fat or water from the image. A "water image" eliminates fat; a "fat image" eliminates water. An "in-phase image" can resemble either T1, T2, and SPGR sequences. IDEAL performs all of these options in one acquisition. Applications include orbits, pituitary, and IACs.
- CUBE (GE) is an isotropic T2 or T2 FLAIR imaging option with sub-millimeter slices and isotropic pixels, which are acquired in the sagittal or coronal plain. These isotropic images can be reformatted into other planes post acquisition. For MS of the brain, the sagittal plane is performed and reformats are acquired in the axial and coronal plane.
- Two-dimensional SWI and three-dimensional SWAN are "susceptibility-weighted imaging," which are more susceptible to blood and or blood vessels. These may replace routine GRE imaging for blood or trauma. They should be reformatted in the axial plane, with minimal rendering, to increase visualization of vessels and blood products.
- Contrast is predominantly used with T1 FSE, T1 FLAIR, BRAVO, and other T1 SPGR sequences because it shortens the T1 relaxation rate and T1 effects are maximized.
- MRA (magnetic resonance angiography) are spoiled gradient and gradient echo sequences that suppress background tissue while enhancing vascular structures by using low TR, low TE, and low flip angles (FA). Saturation bands are used to distinguish between arteries and veins. Above the heart, superior (S) sat bands visualize arteries and inferior (I) sat bands visualize veins. For suspected dissection, always add an axial T1 fat-saturated sequence.
- TOF (time of flight) sequences are 2D or 3D imaging techniques that rely primarily on flow-related enhancement to distinguish moving spins from stationary tissue. Blood that flows into the slice will not have experienced RF pulses saturation and will therefore appear much brighter than stationary tissue.
- PC (phase contrast) imaging sequences use gradient directions and flow Velocity ENCoding (VENC) to visualize arteries and veins based on their speed of flow in cm/sec. Because stationary tissue does not move, it is automatically suppressed.

Vessels are always flowing so they are bright on phase contrast scans. Veins flow slower then arteries at approximately 15-20 cm/sec, whereas arteries flow at approx 50-70 cm/sec.

- Enhanced MRA and MRV are high-resolution PC sequences that can be used to replace TOF imaging. It has the ability to eliminate vascular susceptibility issues that occur with TOF sequences, because it uses the velocity of the flow instead of flow-related enhancement.

Options

- Inferior (I) saturation (sat) band can help to compensate for CSF and vascular pulsation. Vascular structures should have a flow void (appear dark) on T1 and T2 pulse sequences. Saturation bands can be used on all pulse sequences.
- Flow compensation (FC) or gradient nulling should be used on T2 images to help compensate for CSF flow and vascular motion. FC should never be used on T1 pre-contrast because it can cause vessels to appear bright and mimic pathology. It is often used post gadolinium (GAD) on T1 sequences to compensate for flow artefacts.
- Fat saturation (FS) options and terminology are vendor specific. For GE systems, use "fat classic" for fat saturation of the orbits and internal auditory canals.

ROUTINE BRAIN SCAN

Acquire three-plane pilot per site specifications.

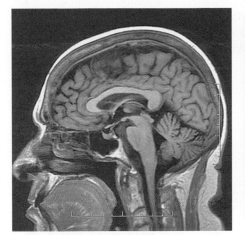

Figure 1-1 Sagittal brain

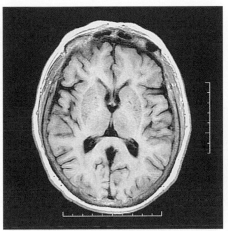

Figure 1-2 Axial brain

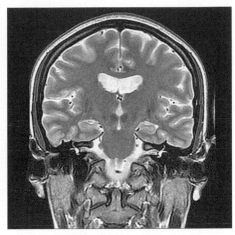

Figure 1-3 Coronal brain

COIL: Multi-channel head or neurovascular*
POSITION: Supine, head first, cushion under knees
LANDMARK: Glabella
IMMOBILIZATION: Secure head with sponges. Shield patient from touching sides of magnet

*Reference safety parameters specific to each coil.

Acquisition of Sagittal Images of the Brain

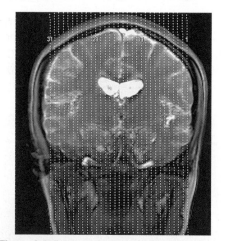

Figure 1-4 Coronal-midline brain with sagittal locs

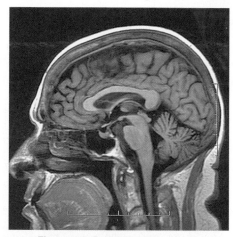

Figure 1-5 Sagittal-midline brain

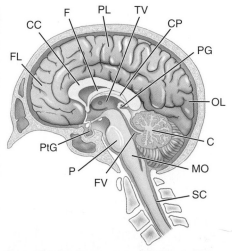

Figure 1-6 Sagittal anatomy-midline brain

SLICE ACQUISITION: Plot left to right covering both temporal margins

SLICE ALIGNMENT: Parallel to third ventricle and midsagittal fissure

ANATOMIC COVERAGE: C2 to convexity, anterior to posterior cranial margins

TIP: Make sure C2 is included in the scanning range to demonstrate best the cerebellum tonsils.

KEY: **C**, cerebellum; **CC**, corpus callosum; **CP**, choroid plexus; **F**, fornix; **FL**, frontal lobe; **FV**, fourth ventricle; **MO**, medulla oblongata; **OL**, occipital lobe; **P**, pons; **PG**, pineal gland; **PL**, parietal lobe; **PtG**, pituitary gland; **SC**, spinal cord; **TV**, third ventricle.

Acquisition of Axial Images of the Brain

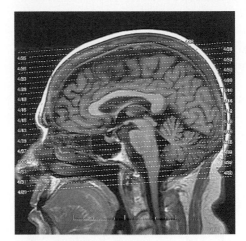

Figure 1-7 Midline sagittal image with axial locs

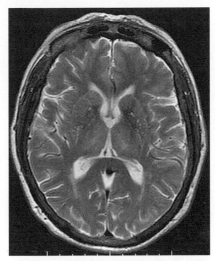

Figure 1-8 Axial image of brain

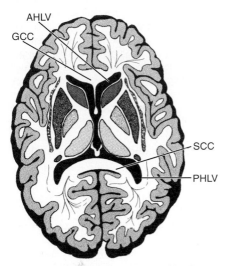

Figure 1-9 Axial anatomy of brain

SLICE ACQUISITION: Plot inferior to superior, foramen magnum to vertex
SLICE ALIGNMENT: Parallel to genu and splenium of corpus callosum
ANATOMIC COVERAGE: Nasion to occiput, cerebellum to vertex covering the cranial margin

KEY: **AHLV**, anterior horn of lateral ventricle; **GCC**, genu of corpus callosum; **PHLV**, posterior horn of lateral ventricle; **SCC**, splenium of corpus callosum.

TIP: Angle to the genu and splenium so that duplication for subsequent examinations is possible.

Acquisition of Coronal Images of the Brain

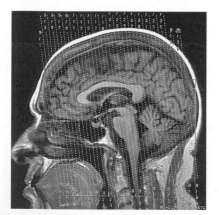

Figure 1-10 Midline sagittal image with coronal locs

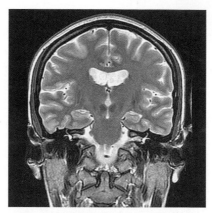

Figure 1-11 Midline coronal image

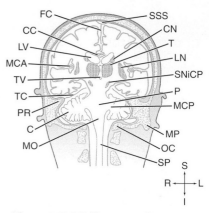

Figure 1-12 Midline coronal anatomy

SLICE ACQUISITION: Plot anterior to the posterior, frontal sinus through occiput, cervical to vertex

SLICE ALIGNMENT: Perpendicular to the genu and splenium of corpus callosum

ANATOMIC COVERAGE: C2 to vertex, covering cranial margins

TIP: Coronals should be acquired with slices angled perpendicular to the corpus callosum to ensure duplication.

KEY: **C**, cerebellum; **CC**, corpus callosum; **CN**, caudate nucleus; **FC**, falx cerebri; **LN**, lentiform nucleus; **LV**, lateral ventricle; **MCA**, middle cerebral artery; **MCP**, middle cerebellar penduncle; **MO**, medulla oblongata; **MP**, mastoid process; **OC**, occipital condyle; **P**, pons; **PR**, petrous ridge; **SNiCP**, substantia nigra in cerebral penduncle; **SP**, spinal cord; **SSS**, superior sagittal sinus; **T**, thalamus; **TC**, tentorium cerebelli; **TV**, third ventricle.

| Table 1-1 | Routine Brain |

Sequence 1.5	TR	TE	ETL or FA	Bandwidth	F Matrix	Ph Matrix	FOV	Slice Thick	Inter-space	NEX	TI	Pulse Sequence Options
Sag. T1 FSE	500	Min	3-4	31.25	320	224	24/24	5	0	1		Sat I
Cor. T2 FSE	4550	102	13	41.67	320	224	22/.75	5	0	2		FC
*Ax. DWI	8000	84		62.5	128	128	22/22	5	0	2		EPI, Diff, Asset, SPF, BV1000
Ax.T2 Flair	8000	135	35	41.67	288	288	22/22	5	0	1.5	2000	FC, Propeller
Ax.T2 FSE	4000	129	27	41.67	320	320	22/22	5	0	1.5		FC, Propeller
Ax SWI	5000	Min	90FA		192	320	22/22	2.4	0	4		EPI, FC, Freq R-L
Post GAD												
Cor. T1 FSE	500	Min	3-4	31.25	320	224	22/.75	5	0	1		Sat I, FC
Sag. T1 FSE	500	Min	3-4	31.25	320	224	24/24	5	0	1		Sat I, FC
Ax. T1 FSE	600	Min	3-4	31.25	256	224	22/.75	5	0	1		Sat I, FC

(Continued)

Table 1-1 | Routine Brain—*cont'd*

Sequence 3T	TR	TE	ETL or FA	Bandwidth	F Matrix	Ph Matrix	FOV	Slice Thick	Inter-space	NEX	TI	Pulse Sequence Options
Sag. T1 Flair	3000	17	10	31.25	288	224	24/24	4	0	1	1200	Sat I, FC, Seq, 2 Acq
Cor. T2	4700	100	14	62.50	288	224	22/.75	4	0	1		FC
Ax. DWI	7000	Min		250	128	192	22/22	5	0	1		EPI, Diff, Asset, SPF, BV 1000
Ax. T2 Flair	9500	132	36	83.33	320	288	22/22	5	0	1.5	2375	FC, Propeller
Ax. T2 FSE	6500	128	32	100	416	288	22/22	5	0	1.5		FC, Prop
Ax T1 Flair	3000	17	10	31.25	288	192	22/22	5	0		1200	FC, Seq, 2 Acq

Table 1-1 Routine Brain—*cont'd*

Sequence 3T	TR	TE	ETL or FA	Bandwidth	F Matrix	Ph Matrix	FOV	Slice Thick	Inter-space	NEX	TI	Pulse Sequence Options
Ax SWI	5000	Min	FA90		192	320	22/22	5	0	4		EPI, FC, Freq R-L
Post GAD												
Cor.T1 SPGR	375	Min		62.50	288	224	22/22	5	0	1		Sat I, FC, Zip 512
Sag.T1 SPGR	375	Min		62.50	288	224	24/24	5	0	1		Sat I, FC, Zip 512
Ax.T1 SPGR	375	Min		62.50	288	224	22/22	5	0	1		Sat I, FC, Zip 512

Angle to anterior (genu) and posterior (splenium) of the corpus callosum. DWI is used for possible stroke, B Value 1000.

Add FLAIR post gadolinium for suspected meningeal disease.

TRF (Tailor Radio-Frequency) should be used with all FSE sequences to increase # of slices per TR.

Prop (Propeller) pulse sequences reduces motion artefacts and should be used when available.

Table 1-2   Site Protocol: Routine Brain

Sequence 1.5	TR	TE	ETL	Bandwidth	F Matrix	Ph Matrix	FOV	Slice Thick	Inter-space	NEX	TI	Pulse Sequence Options
Post GAD												

Sequence 3T	TR	TE	ETL	Bandwidth	F Matrix	Ph Matrix	FOV	Slice Thick	Inter-space	NEX	TI	Pulse Sequence Options
Post GAD												

Table 1-2 Site Protocol: Routine Brain—*cont'd*

BRAIN FOR PITUITARY

Acquire three plane pilot per site specifications (see Figs. 1-1 through 1-3).

Acquisition of Coronal Images, Thin Slices Through Pituitary

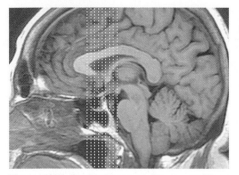

Figure 1-13 Sagittal image with coronal locs for pituitary

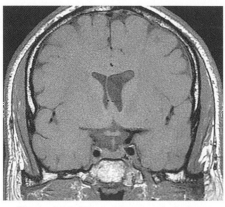

Figure 1-14 Coronal image of pituitary

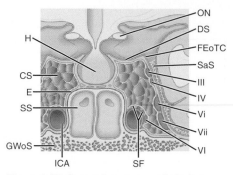

Figure 1-15 Coronal anatomy of pituitary

KEY: **CS**, cavernous sinus; **DS**, diaphragma sellae; **E**, endosteum; **FEoTC**, free edge of tentorium cerebelli; **GWoS**, greater wing of sphenoid; **H**, hypophysis; **ICA**, internal carotid artery; **ON**, optic nerve; **SaS**, subarachnoid space; **SF**, sympathetic fibers; **SS**, sphenoid sinus.

SLICE ACQUISITION: Plot anterior to posterior
SLICE ALIGNMENT: Parallel to sella turcica
ANATOMIC COVERAGE: From anterior corpus callosum through pons, cerebellum to vertex

Acquisition of Sagittal Images of Pituitary

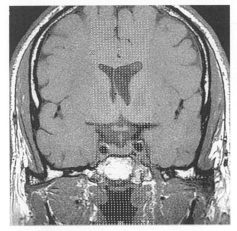

Figure 1-16 Coronal image with thin sagittal locs for pituitary

Figure 1-17 Sagittal midline image of pituitary

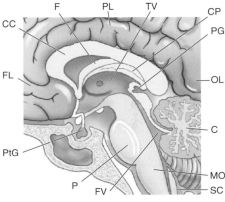

Figure 1-18 Sagittal anatomy of pituitary

SLICE ACQUISITION: Plot left to right
SLICE ALIGNMENT: Parallel to pituitary stalk
ANATOMIC COVERAGE: From left to right internal carotid arteries

KEY: **C**, cerebellum; **CC**, corpus callosum; **CP**, choroid plexus; **F**, fornix; **FL**, frontal lobe; **FV**, fourth ventricle; **MO**, medulla oblongata; **OL**, occipital lobe; **P**, pons; **PG**, pineal gland; **PL**, parietal lobe; **PtG**, pituitary gland; **SC**, spinal cord; **TV**, third ventricle.

Table 1-3 Brain for Pituitary

Sequence 1.5	TR	TE	ETL or FA	Bandwidth	F Matrix	Ph Matrix	FOV	Slice Thick	Inter-space	NEX	TI	Pulse Sequence Options
SagT1	500	Min		31.25	320	224	16/16	3	0	3		SE, Sat I, NPW
Cor T2 FSE	4000	120	27	41.67	320	256	16/16	3	0	2		FC
Cor T1	450	Min		15.63	256	192	16/16	3	0	3		SE, Sat I
OPT T1 COR	400	Min		15.63	256	192	16/16	3	0	1-2		Dynamic 3 slices
Post GAD												
*Cor T1	450	Min		15.63	256	192	14/14	3	.5	3		SE, Sat I, FC
*Sag T1	675	Min		15.63	320	224	18/18	2	.5	2		SE, Sat I, FC, NPW
OPT T1 COR	400	Min		15.63	256	192	16/16	3	0	1-2		Dynamic 3 slices 10-12 times

Table 1-3 Brain for Pituitary—*cont'd*

Sequence 3T	TR	TE	ETL or FA	Band-width	F Matrix	Ph Matrix	FOV	Slice Thick	Inter-space	NEX	TI	Pulse Sequence Options
SagT1 FLAIR	3000	17	10	31.25	288	224	14/14	4	0	1	1200	FC, Sat I, Seq
CorT2 FSE	6500	120	32	62.50	416	416	14/14	4	0	1		FC
Cor T1 FLAIR	3000	17	10	31.25	288	224	14/14	3	0	1	1200	Sat I, FC, Seq
OPT T1 COR	400	Min		15.63	256	192	16/16	3	0	1-2		Dynamic 3 slices 10-12 times
Post GAD												
Cor T1 FLAIR	3000	17	10	31.25	288	224	14/14	3	0	1	1200	Sat I, FC, TRF, Seq
Sag. T1 FLAIR	3000	17	10	31.25	288	224	14/14	2	0	2	1200	Sat I, FC, TRF, NPW, Seq
OPT T1 Cor	400	Min		15.63	256	192	16/16	3	0	1.2		Dynamic 3 slices 10-12 times

T1 FSE can be substituted for T1 SE.
TRF (Tailor Radio-Frequency) should be used with all FSE sequences to increase # of slices per TR.
OPT Dynamic T1 Coronal is scanned multiple times per slice.
Axial T1 should be added post gadolinium for other brain pathology.

Table 1-4   Site Protocol: Pituitary

Sequence 1.5	TR	TE	ETL/ FA	Bandwidth	F Matrix	Ph Matrix	FOV	Slice Thick	Interspace	NEX	TI	Pulse Sequence Options
Post GAD												

Table 1-4   Site Protocol: Pituitary—*cont'd*

Sequence 3T	TR	TE	ETL	Bandwidth	F Matrix	Ph Matrix	FOV	Slice Thick	Interspace	NEX	TI	Pulse Sequence Options
Post GAD												

BRAIN FOR INTERNAL AUDITORY CANALS (IACs)

Acquire three-plane pilot per site specifications (see Figs. 1-1 through 1-3).

Acquisition of Thin-Sliced Axial Images of the IACs

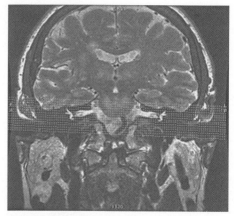

Figure 1-19 Coronal image with thin axial locs for IACs

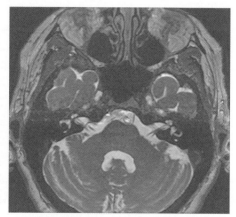

Figure 1-20 Axial image of IACs

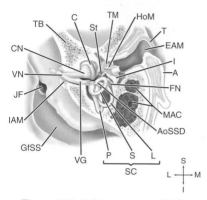

Figure 1-21 Axial anatomy of IACs

KEY: A, auricle (pinna); **AoSSD,** ampulla of superior semicircular duct; **C,** cochlea; **CN,** cochlear nerve (CN VIII); **EAM,** external auditory meatus; **FN,** facial nerve (CN VII) in facial canal; **GfSS,** groove for sigmoid sinus; **HoM,** head of malleus; **I,** incus; **IAM,** internal auditory meatus; **JF,** jugular foramen; **L,** lateral; **MAC,** mastoid air cells; **P,** posterior; **S,** superior (anterior); **SC,** semicircular canals; **St,** stapes. **T,** tragus; **TB,** temporal bone (petrous part); **TM,** tympanic membrane; **VG,** vestibular ganglion; **VN,** vestibular nerve (CN VIII).

SLICE ACQUISITION: Plot inferior to superior
SLICE ALIGNMENT: Parallel to acoustic nerves
ANATOMICAL COVERAGE: From inferior to superior through bony mastoid region

Acquisition of Thin-Sliced Coronal Images of the IACs

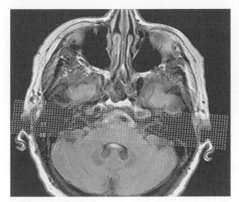

Figure 1-22 Axial image with thin-sliced coronal locs for IACs

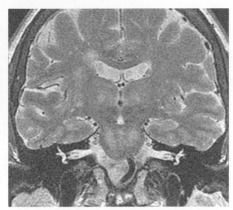

Figure 1-23 Coronal image of IACs

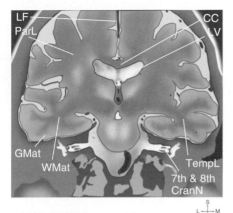

Figure 1-24 Coronal anatomy of IACs

SLICE ACQUISITION: Plot anterior to posterior
SLICE ALIGNMENT: Parallel to IACs
ANATOMIC COVERAGE: Anterior to posterior through bony mastoid region

Key: **CC**, corpus callosum; **GMat**, gray matter; **LF**, longitudinal fissure; **LV**, lateral ventricle; **ParL**, parietal lobe; **TempL**, temporal lobe; **WMat**, white matter; **7th & 8th CranN**, 7th and 8th cranial nerves.

Table 1-5   Brain for IACs

Sequence 1.5	TR	TE	ETL or FA	Band-width	F Matrix	Ph Matrix	FOV	Slice Thick	Inter-space	NEX	TI	Pulse Sequence Options
Sag T1 FSE	500	Min		31.25	320	224	24/24	5	0	1		Sat I
Ax T2 FLAIR	8000	135	35	41.67	288	288	22/22	5	0	1.5	2000	FC, propeller
Cor T2 FSE	4500	102	13	41.67	320	224	18/18	3	0	2		FSE, FC
Ax 3-D Fiesta		Min	FA 45	62.50	448	256	16/16	.8	0	4		Zip 2, loc/slab 40
Ax T1 SE FS	550	Min		15.63	256	224	16/16	3	0	3		Sat I, F
Post GAD												
Ax T1 SE FS	700	Min		15.63	256	224	16/16	3	0	2		Sat I, F, FC
Cor T1 SE FS	675	Min		15.63	320	224	16/16	3	0	2		Sat I, F, FC

Table 1-5 Brain for IACs—*cont'd*

Sequence 3T	TR	TE	ETL or FA	Bandwidth	F Matrix	Ph Matrix	FOV	Slice Thick	Inter-space	NEX	TI	Pulse Sequence Options
Sag T1 Flair	3000	17	10	31.25	288	224	24/24	4	0	1	1200	Sat I, FC, Seq, 2 Acq
Ax.T2 Flair	9500	132	36	83.33	288	288	22/22	5	0	1.5	2375	FC, Propeller
Cor T2	4250	100	18	62.50	320	224	18/18	2	0	2		FC
Ax 3D Fiesta	Mach	Min	FA 45	62.50	512	256	14/14	.8	0	2		Zip 2, Loc/ slab 40
*Ax T1Flair FS	3000	17	10	31.25	288	224	16/16	2	0	2	1200	Fat F, FC, TRF, Seq
Post GAD												
Ax T1Flair FS	3000	17	10	31.25	288	224	16/16	2	0	2	1200	Sat F, FC, Seq
Cor T1Flair	3000	17	10	31.25	288	224	16/16	2	0	2	1200	Sat F, FC, Seq

T1 Ax, Cor and 3D Fiesta (Steady State) scan through the IAC's only.
T1 FSE can be substituted for T1 SE.
TRF (Tailor Radio-Frequency) should be used with all FSE and Flair sequences to increase # of slices per TR.
Prop (Propeller) Pulse sequence reduces motion artefacts and should be used when available.

Table 1-6 Site Protocol: IAC

Sequence 1.5	TR	TE	ETL/ FA	Bandwidth	F Matrix	Ph Matrix	FOV	Slice Thick	Interspace	NEX	TI	Pulse Sequence Options
Post GAD												

Table 1-6	Site Protocol: IAC—*cont'd*												
Sequence 3T	TR	TE	ETL/ FA	Bandwidth	F Matrix	Ph Matrix	FOV	Slice Thick	Interspace	NEX	TI	Pulse Sequence Options
Post GAD												

BRAIN FOR ORBITS—OPTIC NERVES

Acquire three-plane pilots per site specifications (see Figs. 1-1 through 1-3).

Acquisition of Coronal Images of Orbits and Optic Nerves

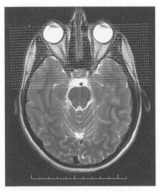

Figure 1-25 Axial brain with thin-sliced coronal locs

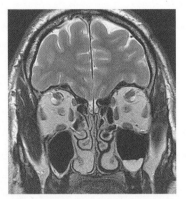

Figure 1-26 Coronal image of IACs

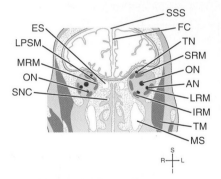

Figure 1-27 Coronal anatomy

SLICE ACQUISITION: Plot anterior to posterior
SLICE ALIGNMENT: Perpendicular to bilateral zygomas
ANATOMIC COVERAGE: From globe of eye through optic chiasm

KEY: **AN**, abducens nerve; **ES**, ethmoid sinus; **FC**, falx cerebri; **IRM**, inferior rectus muscle; **LPSM**, levator palpebrae superioris muscle; **LRM**, lateral rectus muscle; **MRM**, medial rectus muscle; **MS**, maxillary sinus; **ON**, oculomotor nerve; **ON**, optic nerve; **SNC**, superior nasal concha; **SRM**, superior rectus muscle; **SSS**, superior sagittal sinus; **TM**, temporalis muscle; **TN**, trochlear nerve.

TIP: Remove contacts and all eye makeup (makeup causes artifacts). Use caution when scanning patients with tattooed eyeliner.

Acquisition of Axial Images of Orbits and Optic Nerves

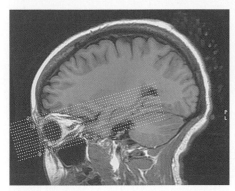

Figure 1-28 Parasagittal image of brain with axial locs

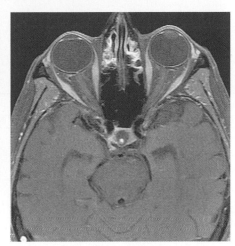

Figure 1-29 Axial image of orbits-optic nerves

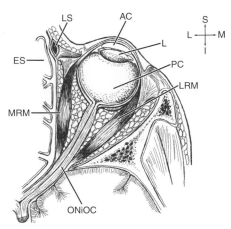

Figure 1-30 Axial anatomy

KEY: **AC**, anterior compartment; **ES**, ethmoid sinus; **L**, lens; **LRM**, lateral rectus muscle; **LS**, lacrimal sac; **MRM**, medial rectus muscle; **ONiOC**, optic nerve in optic canal; **PC**, posterior compartment.

SLICE ACQUISITION: Plot inferior to superior, on parasagittal slice

SLICE ALIGNMENT: Parallel to optic nerve

ANATOMIC COVERAGE: Inferior to superior orbital margins, globe through posterior cerebellum

Table 1-7 Brain for Orbits

Sequence 1.5	TR	TE	ETL/ FA	Band-width	F Matrix	Ph Matrix	FOV	Slice Thick	Inter-space	NEX	TI	Pulse Sequence Options
Sag T1 SE	500	Min		31.25	320	224	24/24	5	0	1		Sat I
Ax T2 Flair	8000	135	35	41.67	288	288	22/22	5	0	1.5	2000	FC, Propeller
CorT2 FRFSE FS	4500	102	13	41.67	320	224	18/18	4	0	3		Sat F, FC
Ax T1 SE FS	550	Min		15.63	256	224	16/16	3	0	3		Sat F, NPW
Post GAD												
Ax T1 SE FS	550	Min		15.63	256	224	16/16	3	0	3		Sat F, FC, NPW
Cor T1 SE FS	450	Min		115.63	320	224	18/18	4	.5	2		Sat F, FC

| Table 1-7 | Brain for Orbits—*cont'd* | | | | | | | | | | | |

Sequence 3T	TR	TE	ETL/ FA	Bandwidth	F Matrix	Ph Matrix	FOV	Slice Thick	Inter-space	NEX	TI	Pulse Sequence Options
Sag T1 Flair	3000	17	10	31.25	288	224	24/24	4	0	1	1200	Sat I, FC, Seq, 2 Acq
Ax.T2 Flair	9500	132	36	83.33	288	288	22/22	5	0	1.5	2375	FC, Propeller
Cor T2 FRFSE FS	3500	102	17	50.00	416	224	16/16	3	0	2		Sat F, FC
Ax T1Flair FS	3000	17	10	31.25	288	224	16/16	3	0	1	1200	Sat F, Seq, NPW
Post GAD												
Ax T1 Flair FS	3000	17	10	31.25	288	224	16/16	3	0	1	1200	Sat F, FC, Seq, NPW
CorT1 Flair FS	3000	17	10	31.25	288	224	16/16	3	0	2	1200	Sat F, FC, Seq

Ax FLAIR scan through the brain.
Coronal thin slices to include the Optic Chiasm.
T1 FSE can be substituted for T1 SE.
TRF (Tailor Radio-Frequency) should be used with all FSE and Flair sequences to increase # of slices per TR.
Prop (Propeller) Pulse sequence reduces motion artefacts and should be used when available.

Table 1-8 Site Protocol: Orbits

Sequence 1.5	TR	TE	ETL/ FA	Bandwidth	F Matrix	Ph Matrix	FOV	Slice Thick	Interspace	NEX	TI	Pulse Sequence Options
Post GAD												

Table 1-8 Site Protocol: Orbits—*cont'd*

Sequence 3T	TR	TE	ETL/ FA	Bandwidth	F Matrix	Ph Matrix	FOV	Slice Thick	Interspace	NEX	TI	Pulse Sequence Options
Post GAD												

BRAIN FOR MULTIPLE SCLEROSIS

Acquire three-plane pilot per site specifications (see Figs. 1-1 through 1-3).

Acquisition of Thin Sagittal Images

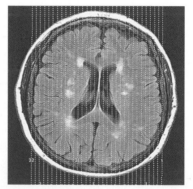

Figure 1-31 Axial image with thin sagittal locs

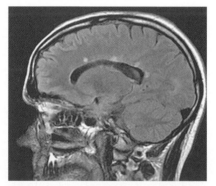

Figure 1-32 Sagittal image with plaques

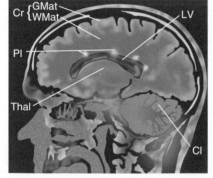

Figure 1-33 Sagittal anatomy

SLICE ACQUISITION: Plot left to right, covering both temporal margins
SLICE ALIGNMENT: Parallel to third ventricle and midsagittal fissure
ANATOMIC COVERAGE: Anterior to posterior cranial margins, C2 to vertex

KEY: **Cl**, cerebellum; **Cr**, Cerebrum; **GMat**, gray matter; **LV**, lateral ventricle; **Pl**, plaque; **Thal**, thalamus; **WMat**, white matter.

TIP: When performing comparison studies, matching the field of view, slice thickness, and field strength should be considered.

Table 1-9 Brain for Multiple Sclerosis

Sequence 1.5	TR	TE	ETL or FA	Band-width	F Matrix	Ph Matrix	FOV	Slice Thick	Inter-space	NEX	TI	Pulse Sequence Options
Sag T2Flair	8800	130		31.25	256	224	24/24	4	0	1	2200	FC
Ax DWI	8000	84		62.5	128	128	22/22	5	0	2		EPI, Diff, Asset, SPF, BV1000
Ax T2 Flair	8000	135	35	41.67	288	288	22/22	5	0	1.5	2000	FC, Propeller
Ax T2 FSE	4000	120	27	41.67	320	320	22/22	5	0	1.5		FC, Propeller
Ax T1 FSE	600	Min	3-4	31.25	256	224	22/.75	5	0	1		Sat I
Post GAD												
Ax T1	600	Min		31.25	256	224	22/.75	5	0	1		SE, Sat I, FC
Cor T1	500	Min		31.25	256	224	22/.75	5	0	1		SE, Sat I, FC
Sag T1	500	Min		31.25	320	224	24/24	4	0	1		SE, Sat I, FC
OPT Ax T1	600	Min		31.25	256	224	22/.75	5	0	1		SE, FC, MgT delayed

(Continued)

Table 1-9 Brain for Multiple Sclerosis—*cont'd*

Sequence 3T	TR	TE	ETL or FA	Band-width	F Matrix	Ph Matrix	FOV	Slice Thick	Inter-space	NEX	TI	Pulse Sequence Options
Sag T2Flair	9000	115		50	384	224	24/24	4	0	1	2375	FC
Ax DWI	7000	min		250	128	192	22/22	5	0	1		EPI, Diff, Asset, SPF, BV 1000
Ax.T2 FSE	6500	128	32	100	416	288	22/22	5	0	1.5		FC, Propeller
Ax T1 Flair	3000	17	10	31.25	288	192	22/22	5	0		1200	FC, Seq, Zip 1025, 2 Acq
Post GAD												
Cor T1	375	Min		62.5	288	224	22/22	5	0	1		FSPGR, Sat I, FC, Zip 512
Sag T1	375	Min	F	62.5	288	224	22/22	5	0	1		FSPGR, Sat I, FC, Zip 512
Ax T1	375	Min	F	62.5	288	224	22/22	5	0	1		FSPGR, Sat I, FC, Zip 512

Magnetization Transfer (MgT) is often indicated in patients with MS to better visualize plaques. Presently is not available at 3T.

CUBE (GE isotropic) T2 Flair sagittal should be performed when available (See grab bag). Reformat images in the axial and coronal plane.

T1 FSE can be substituted for T1 SE.

TRF (Tailor Radio-Frequency) should be used with all FSE and Flair sequences to increase # of slices per TR.

Table 1-10 Site Protocol: Brain for Multiple Sclerosis

Sequence 1.5	TR	TE	ETL/ FA	Bandwidth	F Matrix	Ph Matrix	FOV	Slice Thick	Interspace	NEX	TI	Pulse Sequence Options
Post GAD												

(Continued)

Table 1-10 Site Protocol: Brain for Multiple Sclerosis—*cont'd*

Sequence 3T	TR	TE	ETL/ FA	Bandwidth	F Matrix	Ph Matrix	FOV	Slice Thick	Interspace	NEX	TI	Pulse Sequence Options
Post GAD												

BRAIN FOR EPILEPSY—TEMPORAL LOBE

Acquisition of Coronal Images

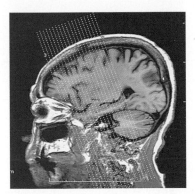

Figure 1-34 Parasagittal image with coronal locs

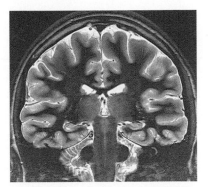

Figure 1-35 Coronal of temporal lobe

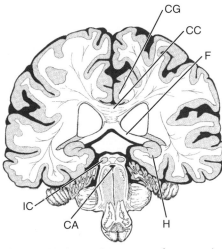

Figure 1-36 Coronal anatomy of temporal lobe

SLICE ACQUISITION: Plot anterior to posterior
SLICE ALIGNMENT: Angled perpendicular to the hippocampus
ANATOMIC COVERAGE: From posterior orbit to include the splenium referenced on axial pilot

> **TIP:** Temporal lobe sequences are plotted off a parasagittal slice, perpendicular to the hippocampus. The splenium can be cross-referenced on the axial pilot. This study can be accompanied by a MRI of the entire brain.

> **KEY: CA**, cerebral aqueduct; **CC**, corpus callosum; **CG**, cingulate gyrus; **F**, fornix; **H**, hippocampus; **IC**, inferior colliculi.

Table 1-11	Brain for Epilepsy: Temporal Lobe

Sequence 1.5	TR	TE	ETL / FA	Bandwidth	F Matrix	Ph Matrix	FOV	Slice Thick	Interspace	NEX	TI	Pulse Sequence Options
Sag. T1	500	Min	3-4	31.25	320	224	24/24	5	0	1		FSE, Sat I
CorT2 FLAIR	8800	120		31.25	256	256	20/20	4	0	1	2200	FC, FAST
CorT2 FSE IR	6000	102	11	41	512	512	20/7.5	3	0	2		FC, FAST
Cor 3D T1		Min	FA 12	15.63	256	256	16/16	1.4	LOCS/slab 136	1	450	3D SPGR, IP prep
Ax.T2 FLAIR	8000	135	35	41.67	288	288	22/22	5	0	1.5	2000	FC, Propeller

Table 1-11 Brain for Epilepsy: Temporal Lobe—*cont'd*

Sequence 3T	TR	TE	ETL/ FA	Bandwidth	F Matrix	Ph Matrix	FOV	Slice Thick	Inter-space	NEX	TI	Pulse Sequence Options
Sag T1 FLAIR	3000	17	10	31.25	288	224	24/24	4	0	1	1200	FC, Seq, TRF
Cor T2 FLAIR	9000	120		31.25	384	224	20/20	4	0	1	2400	FC
Cor FSE IR	4600	40	40	41.67	512	512	20/.75	4	0	2	400	FC, Seq
Cor 3D T1		Min	FA 12	50	256	256	16/16	1.2	LOCS/ slab 136	1	500	3D SPGR, IP Prep
Ax.T2 FLAIR	9500	132	36	83.33	288	288	22/22	5	0	1.5	2375	FC, Propeller

Scan the sagittal through the entire brain.
Angle the coronal to temporal lobe (long axis of hippocampus).
Cor 3D T1 – Scan from the nasion to splenium. Images can be reformatted in the axial plane.

Table 1-12 Site Protocol: Brain for Epilepsy: Temporal Lobe

Sequence 1.5	TR	TE	ETL/ FA	Bandwidth	F Matrix	Ph Matrix	FOV	Slice Thick	Interspace	NEX	TI	Pulse Sequence Options
Post GAD												

Sequence 3T	TR	TE	ETL/ FA	Bandwidth	F Matrix	Ph Matrix	FOV	Slice Thick	Interspace	NEX	TI	Pulse Sequence Options
Post GAD												

Table 1-12 Site Protocol: Brain for Epilepsy: Temporal Lobe—*cont'd*

BRAIN FOR TEMPOROMANDIBULAR JOINTS

Acquire three-plane pilot per site specifications (see Figs. 1-1 through 1-3).

Acquisition of Axial Location Through Mandibular Condyles

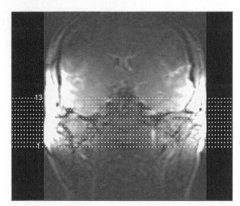

Figure 1-37 Coronal image with axial locs through mandibular condyles

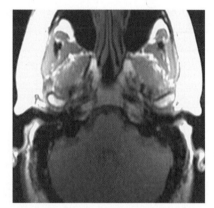

Figure 1-38 Axial image of mandibular condyles

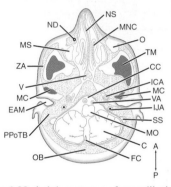

Figure 1-39 Axial anatomy of mandibular condyles

KEY: C, cerebellum; **CC,** cerebellomedullary cistern; **EAM,** external auditory meatus; **FC,** falx cerebelli; **ICA,** internal carotid artery; **IJA,** internal jugular vein; **MC,** mandibular condyles; **MNC,** middle nasal concha; **MO,** medulla oblongata; **MS,** maxillary sinus; **ND,** nasolacrimal duct; **NS,** nasal septum; **O,** orbit; **OB,** occipital bone; **PPoTB,** petrous portion of temporal bone; **SS,** sigmoid sinus; **TM,** temporalis muscle; **V,** vomer; **VA,** vertebral artery; **ZA,** zygomatic arch.

COIL: Bilateral 3-inch coils at 1.5 T (multi-channel head coil may be used if necessary); at 3T, multi-channel head coil is used

SLICE ACQUISITION: Plot inferior to superior

SLICE ALIGNMENT: Perpendicular to mandibular condyloid process

ANATOMIC COVERAGE: From superior rami of mandible through temporal bone

Acquisition of Sagittal Images of Temporomandibular Joints

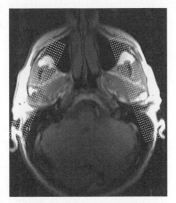

Figure 1-40 Axial image of mandibular condyles with parasagittal locs for TMJs

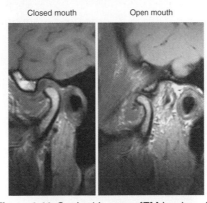

Closed mouth   Open mouth

Figure 1-41 Sagittal image of TMJ—closed mouth

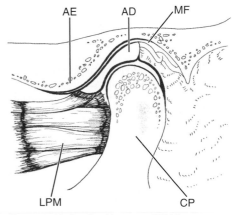

AE   AD   MF

LPM   CP

Figure 1-42 Sagittal image of TMJ—open mouth

SLICE ACQUISITION: Plot each side separately. Plot right side lateral to medial; plot left side lateral to medial

SLICE ALIGNMENT: Perpendicular to mandibular condyles

ANATOMIC COVERAGE: From zygomatic process to temporal bone, lateral to medial (see reference image).

KEY: **AD**, articular disk (meniscus); **AE**, articular eminence; **CP**, condyloid process (condyle of mandible); **LPM**, lateral pterygoid muscle; **MF**, mandibular fossa.

TIP: To obtain open-mouth images, repeat last sagittal sequence with appliance in between the patient's teeth to maintain the jaw in open position while scanning. Ask the patient to open his or her mouth before scanning to see how far the mouth can be opened comfortably. A plastic 10-mL syringe wrapped in sterile gauze and tape is suggested when an appliance is not available.

Acquisition of Coronal Images of Temporomandibular Joints

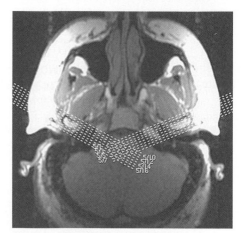

Figure 1-43 Axial image of mandibular condyles with coronal locs for TMJs

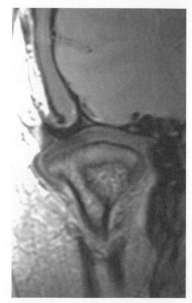

Figure 1-44 Coronal image of TMJ

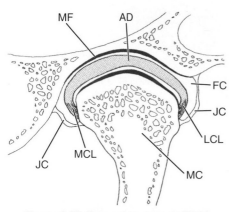

Figure 1-45 Coronal anatomy of TMJ

KEY: **AD**, articular disk (meniscus); **FC**, fibrous capsule; **JC**, joint capsule; **LCL**, lateral collateral ligament; **MC**, mandibular condyle; **MCL**, medial collateral ligament; **MF**, mandibular fossa.

SLICE ACQUISITION: Plot each side separately, anterior to posterior
SLICE ALIGNMENT: Angle slices parallel with TMJ space
ANATOMIC COVERAGE: From zygomatic process through temporal bone

Table 1-13				Temporomandibular Joints									
Sequence 1.5	TR	TE	ETL / FA	Bandwidth	F Matrix	Ph Matrix	FOV	Slice Thick	Interspace	NEX	TI	Pulse Sequence Options
Ax loc	600	M	4	20.83	256	160	24/24	2	0	1		TRF
Sag T1	450	M	3	20.83	256	224	12/12	2	0	4		NPW, TRF, closed
Sag PD	1500	24	7	20.83	320	320	12/12	2	0	3		NPW, TRF
Sag T2 FS	2800	85	16	20.83	256	224	12/12	2	0	4		TRF, NPW, Sat F
Cor PD	1500	24	7	20.83	256	224	12/12	2	0	3		TRF, NPW
Sag T1	450	M	3	20.83	256	224	12/12	2	0	4		TRF, NPW-open

(Continued)

Table 1-13 Temporomandibular Joints—*cont'd*

Sequence 3T	TR	TE	ETL / FA	Band-width	F Matrix	Ph Matrix	FOV	Slice Thick	Interspace	NEX	TI	Pulse Sequence Options
Ax loc	3000	17	10	31.25	256	224	16/16	3	0	1	1200	TRF, Seq
Sag T1	3000	17	10	50	320	224	12/12	2	0	4	1200	TRF, NPW, Seq -closed
Sag PD	3000	30	7	50	320	224	12/12	2	0	3		TRF, NPW, FC
Sag T2 FS	3800	65	15	50	256	224	12/12	2	0	4		TRF, NPW, FC, Sat F
Cor PD	3000	30	7	50	320	224	12/12	2	0	3		TRF, NPW, FC
Sag T1	3000	17	10	50	320	224	12/12	2	0	4	1200	TRF, NPW, Seq open

Can use vendor specific 3" coils or multi-channel head coil.

Table 1-14 Site Protocol: Temporomandibular Joints

Sequence 1.5	TR	TE	ETL/ FA	Bandwidth	F Matrix	Ph Matrix	FOV	Slice Thick	Interspace	NEX	TI	Pulse Sequence Options

(Continued)

Table 1-14 Site Protocol: Temporomandibular Joints—*cont'd*

Sequence 3T	TR	TE	ETL/ FA	Bandwidth	F Matrix	Ph Matrix	FOV	Slice Thick	Interspace	NEX	TI	Pulse Sequence Options

MRA—CIRCLE OF WILLIS

Acquire three-plane pilot per site specifications (see Figs. 1-1 through 1-3).

Acquire a coronal vascular loc per specifications in Table 1-15.

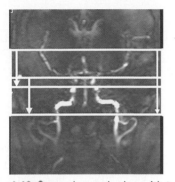

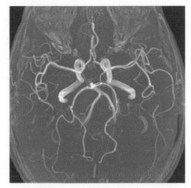

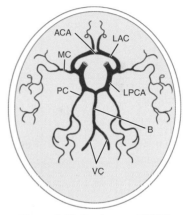

Figure 1-46 Coronal vascular loc with two overlapping slabs

Figure 1-47 Two-dimensional image of COW

Figure 1-48 Anatomy of COW

SLICE ACQUISITION: Plot superior to inferior

ANATOMIC COVERAGE: From vertebral basilar junction to superior COW, at level of lateral ventricle

KEY: **ACA**, anterior communicating artery; **B**, basilar; **LAC**, left anterior cerebral; **LPCA**, left posterior communicating artery; **MC**, middle cerebral; **PC**, posterior cerebral.

TIP: Use the coronal PC location and prescribe slab superior to inferior. Cover from above COW (lateral ventricle) to vertebral-basilar junction, which should be seen on the PC localizer. Vendor-specific time-resolved imaging should be used when injecting contrast. Use a temporal resolution of 3-4 seconds and 15 phases to image arterial and venous visualization of the Circle of Willis and carotid and vertebral vessels.

Table 1-15 MRA of Circle of Willis

Sequence 1.5	TR	TE	ETL/ FA	Bandwidth	F Matrix	Ph Matrix	FOV	Slice Thick	Inter-space	NEX	TI	Pulse Sequence Options
Ax. DWI	8000	84		62.5	128	128	22/22	5	0	2		SE, EPI, Diff, Asset, SPF, BV1000
Cor 2-D PC VAS	25	Min	FA 30	15.63	256	224	22.22	60	0	4		FC, VAS, vol 60
*Ax 3D TOF, 2 slab	30	Min	FA 20	15.63	256	224	22/.81	1.4	36 locs 9mm overlap	—		SPGR TOF, sat S, FC, MgT, ZIP2, ZIP 512, RAMP I/P/L, Projections 19
Post GAD												
Cor. 3-D TRICKS		Min	FA 30	31.25	256	160	24/.7	4		1		ZIP 512, ZIP 2, temp resol 3-4, Scan 15-18 Phases

Table 1-15 MRA of Circle of Willis—*cont'd*

Sequence 3T	TR	TE	ETL/ FA	Bandwidth	F Matrix	Ph Matrix	FOV	Slice Thick	Inter-space	NEX	TI	Pulse Sequence Options
Ax DWI	7000	Min		250	128	192	22/22	5	0			SE, EPI, Diff, Asset, SPF, BV1000
Cor 2D PC VAS	18		FA 15	15.63	256	128	26/.75	50	0	2		FC, VAS, vol 30, phase diff, All directions
*Ax 3-D T O F 3 slab	26	Min	FA 20	31.25	512	256	22/.88	1.2	36 locs 9mm overlap			SPGR TOF, sat S, FC, MgT, ZIP2, RAMP IS, Projections 19
Post GAD												
Cor 3-D TRICKS		Min	FA 30	125	256	256	26/.27	4		1		ZIP 2, ZIP 512, temp resol 3-4, Scan 15-18 Phases

Use the coronal PC loc to best visualize vessels. Cover from above COW (Lateral Ventricle) to Vertebral-Basilar junction.
Prescribe slab superior to inferior, using 3 slabs with a 9mm overlap. Use a (S) Superior Sat Band.
MIP the anterior and posterior circulation separately tilting and rotating 180 degrees.
Enhanced PC MRA can be used to replace TOF when available (see grab bag).
Add DWI if MRA is not scanned with a MRI of the brain.

Table 1-16 Site Protocol: Circle of Willis

Sequence 1.5	TR	TE	ETL/ FA	Bandwidth	F Matrix	Ph Matrix	FOV	Slice Thick	Interspace	NEX	TI	Pulse Sequence Options
Post GAD												

Table 1-16 Site Protocol: Circle of Willis—*cont'd*

Sequence 3T	TR	TE	ETL/ FA	Bandwidth	F Matrix	Ph Matrix	FOV	Slice Thick	Interspace	NEX	TI	Pulse Sequence Options
Loc.	Soft	ware	specific	3plane	Loc-	use	asset	calibra	Tion			
Post GAD												
Ax.T1												
Sag.T1												
Cor.T1												

MRV—SUPERIOR SAGITTAL SINUS

Acquire three-plane pilot per site specifications (see Figs. 1-1 through 1-3).

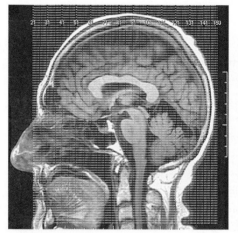

Figure 1-49 Sagittal image with coronal loc

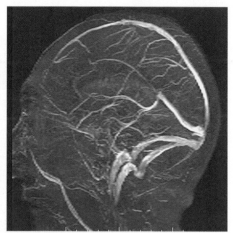

Figure 1-50 Venous image of sagittal sinus

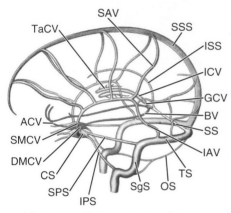

Figure 1-51 Venous anatomy of brain

SLICE ACQUISITION: Plot anterior to posterior
SLICE ALIGNMENT: Do not angle slices
ANATOMIC COVERAGE: Frontal bone to occiput, including bony anatomy

TIP: Scan anterior to posterior outside the cranial margins to avoid clipping vessels.

KEY: **ACV**, anterior cerebral vein; **BV**, basal vein; **CS**, cavernous sinus; **DMCV**, deep middle cerebral vein; **GCV**, great cerebral vein; **IAV**, inferior anastomotic vein; **ICV**, internal cerebral vein; **IPS**, inferior petrosal sinus; **ISS**, inferior sagittal sinus; **OS**, occipital sinus; **SAV**, superior anastomotic vein. **SgS**, sigmoid sinus; **SMCV**, superficial middle cerebral vein; **SPS**, superior petrosal sinus; **SS**, straight sinus; **SSS**, superior sagittal sinus; **TaCV**, thalamostriate and choroidal veins; **TS**, transverse sinus.

Table 1-17 MRV—Sagittal Sinus

Sequence 1.5	TR	TE	ETL / FA	Bandwidth	F Matrix	Ph Matrix	FOV	Slice Thick	Inter-space	NEX	TI	Pulse Sequence Options
Ax. DWI	8000	84		62.5	128	128	22/22	5	0	2		SE, EPI, diff, asset, SPF, BV1000
Cor 2-D PC VAS	25	Min	FA 30	15.63	256	224	22.22	60	0	4		FC, VAS, Vol 60
Cor TOF	26	Min	FA 60	31.25	256	224	24/.75	1.5	0	1		VAS TOF SPGR Sat I, FC, Seq, Projection 1

(Continued)

Table 1-17 MRV—Sagittal Sinus—*cont'd*

Sequence 3T	TR	TE	ETL/ FA	Bandwidth	F Matrix	Ph Matrix	FOV	Slice Thick	Inter- space	NEX	TI	Pulse Sequence Options
Ax. DWI	7000	Min		250	128	192	22/22	5	0	1		SE, EPI, diff, Asset, SPF, BV1000
Cor 2-D PC VAS	18		FA 15	15.63	256	128	26/.75	50	0	2		FC, VAS, vol 30 Phase Diff, All Directions, 19 Projections
Cor TOF	Min	Min	FA 70	31.25	320	192	22/.75	1.5	0	1		VAS TOF, Sat I, FC, Seq

Scan from anterior cranium to posterior cranium to avoid clipping the vessels.
Use a (I) Inferior Sat Band.
MIP the coronal 2D TOF, rotating laterally 180 degrees.
Use Enhanced PC MRA when available (see grab bag).
Add DWI if MRA is not scanned with a MRI of the brain.

Table 1-18 Site Protocol: MRV—Sagittal Sinus

Sequence 1.5	TR	TE	ETL/ FA	Bandwidth	F Matrix	Ph Matrix	FOV	Slice Thick	Interspace	NEX	TI	Pulse Sequence Options

(Continued)

Table 1-18 Site Protocol: MRV—Sagittal Sinus—*cont'd*

Sequence 3T	TR	TE	ETL/ FA	Bandwidth	F Matrix	Ph Matrix	FOV	Slice Thick	Interspace	NEX	TI	Pulse Sequence Options

BRAIN FOR CEREBROSPINAL FLUID

Acquire three-plane pilot per site specifications (see Figs. 1-1 through 1-3).

Acquisition of Sagittal Image

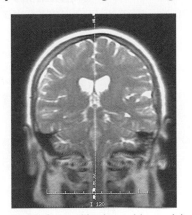

Figure 1-52 Coronal brain—mid ventricles sagittal loc for CSF flow

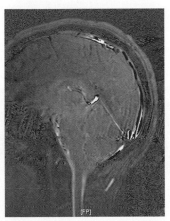

Figure 1-53 Sagittal image—single shot to demonstrate CSF flow

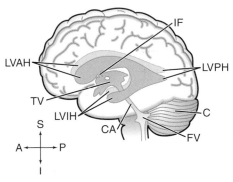

Figure 1-54 Sagittal anatomy for CSF

KEY: C, cerebellum; **CA**, cerebral aqueduct (of Sylvius); **FV**, fourth ventricle; **IF**, interventricular foramen (of Monro); **LVAH**, lateral ventricles, anterior horns; **LVIH**, lateral ventricles, inferior horns; **LVPH**, lateral ventricles, posterior horns; **TV**, third ventricle.

COIL: Multi-channel head or multi-channel neurovascular coil
SLICE ACQUISITION: Single midline slice
SLICE ALIGNMENT: Parallel to and through the fourth ventricle and interhemispheric fissure
ANATOMIC COVERAGE: Brainstem to vertex

TIP: Put peripheral gating probe on the patient before positioning the patient. Make sure gating is working properly.

Acquisition of Axial Image

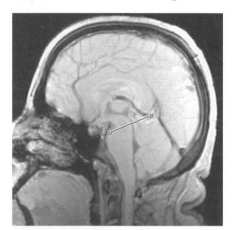

Figure 1-55 Inverted midline sagittal image with loc for single slice through the aqueduct of Sylvius

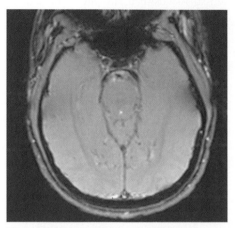

Figure 1-56 Axial image of cerebrospinal fluid flow in the aqueduct of Sylvius

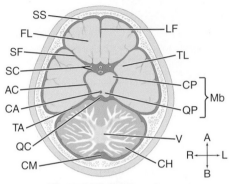

Figure 1-57 Axial anatomy

SLICE ACQUISITION: Single axial slice through aqueduct of Sylvius
SLICE ALIGNMENT: Perpendicular to aqueduct of Sylvius
ANATOMIC COVERAGE: Sphenoid sinus through occiput

TIP: Aqueduct can be seen on the sagittal CSF magnitude image.

KEY: **AC**, ambient cistern; **CA**, cerebral aqueduct; **CH**, cerebellar hemisphere; **CM**, cisterna magna; **CP**, cerebral peduncle; **FL**, frontal lobe; **LF**, longitudinal fissure; **Mb**, midbrain; **QC**, quadrigeminal cistern; **QP**, quadrigeminal plate; **SC**, suprasellar cistern; **SF**, sylvian fissure; **SS**, subarachnoid space; **TA**, tentorial attachment; **TL**, temporal lobe; **V**, vermis.

Table 1-19 Brain for Cerebrospinal Fluid

Sequence 1.5	TR	TE	ETL/ FA	Bandwidth	F Matrix	Ph Matrix	FOV	Slice Thick	Inter-space	NEX	TI	Pulse Sequence Options
Sag CSF flow	38	Mach	FA 20	15.63	256	192	24	5	0	2		Cine, Vas PC, FC, Seq, 4 Flow Phase Diff, Flow All, Flow Velocity 5cm/sec, # phase 32/1 Loc PG Gated, Flow Analysis off, NPW
Ax CSF flow	38	Mach	FA 20	15.63	256	192	24	5	0	2		Cine, Vas PC, FC, Seq, 4 Flow Phase Diff, Flow All, Flow Velocity 5cm/sec, # phase 32/1 Loc PG Gated, Flow Analysis off, NPW

(Continued)

61

Table 1-19 Brain for Cerebrospinal Fluid—*cont'd*

Sequence 3T	TR	TE	ETL/ FA	Band-width	F Matrix	Ph Matrix	FOV	Slice Thick	Inter-space	NEX	TI	Pulse Sequence Options
Sag CSF flow	38	Mach	FA 20	15.63	256	192	24	5	0	2		Cine, Vas PC, FC, Seq, 4 Flow Phase Diff, Flow All, Flow Velocity 5 cm/sec, # phase 32/1 Loc PG Gated, Flow Analysis off, NPW
Ax CSF flow	38	Mach	FA 20	15.63	256	192	24	5	0	2		Cine, Vas PC, FC, Seq, 4 Flow Phase Diff, Flow All, Flow Velocity 5cm/sec, # phase 32/1 Loc PG Gated, Flow Analysis off, NPW

CSF Flow needs PG (peripheral gating). Make sure PG is working properly.

Table 1-20 Site Protocol: Cerebrospinal Fluid

Sequence 1.5	TR	TE	ETL/ FA	Bandwidth	F Matrix	Ph Matrix	FOV	Slice Thick	Interspace	NEX	TI	Pulse Sequence Options
Post GAD												

(Continued)

Table 1-20 Site Protocol: Cerebrospinal Fluid—*cont'd*

Sequence 3T	TR	TE	ETL/ FA	Bandwidth	F Matrix	Ph Matrix	FOV	Slice Thick	Interspace	NEX	TI	Pulse Sequence Options
Loc.	Soft	ware	specific	3plane	Loc-	use	asset	calibra	Tion			
Post GAD												
Ax.T1												
Sag.T1												
Cor.T1												

BRAIN FOR STROKE

Acquire three-plane pilot per site specifications (see Figs. 1-1 through 1-3).

Acquisition of Axial Image

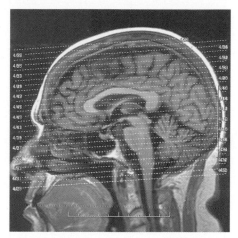

Figure 1-58 Sagittal image with axial locs

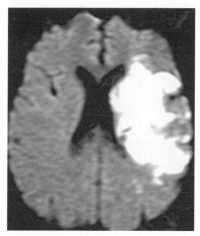

Figure 1-59 Axial image of brain post stroke

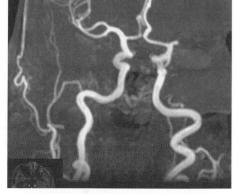

Figure 1-60 MRA COW post stroke

COIL: Multi-channel head or eight-channel neurovascular
SLICE ACQUISITION: Plot inferior to superior, foramen magnum to vertex
SLICE ALIGNMENT: Parallel to genu and splenium of corpus callosum
ANATOMIC COVERAGE: Nasion to occiput, cerebellum to vertex covering cranial margin

> **TIP:** DWI is the most important scan for stroke. It should be performed immediately following the pilot.

Table 1-21 Quick Stroke

Sequence 1.5	TR	TE	ETL	Bandwidth	F Matrix	Ph Matrix	FOV	Slice Thick	Inter-space	NEX	TI	Pulse Sequence Options
Loc.	Soft	ware	specific	3plane	Loc-	use	asset	calibra	Tion			
Ax. DWI	8000	84		62.5	128	128	22/22	5	0	2		SE, EPI, Diff, Asset, SPF, BV1000
Ax. DWI	8000	84		62.5	128	128	22/22	5	0	2		SE, EPI, Diff, Asset, SPF, BV2000
Ax.T2 FLAIR	8000	135	35	41.67	288	288	22/22	5	0	1.5	2000	FC, TRF, Propeller
Ax SWI	5000	Min	90 FA		192	320	22/22	2.4	0	4		EPI, FC, Freg R-1
Post GAD												
Ax Perfusion	2000	Min	FA60		96	128	22/22	7	0	1		GRE, MPh, EPI, 1 shot, Ramp Sampling On, 40 Locs/slice, Interleave

Table 1-21 Quick Stroke—*cont'd*

Sequence 3T	TR	TE	ETL	Band-width	F Matrix	Ph Matrix	FOV	Slice Thick	Interspace	NEX	TI	Pulse Sequence Options
Loc.	Soft	ware	specific	3plane	Loc	use	asset	calibra	tion			
Ax. DWI	7000	min		250	128	192	22/22	5	0	1		SE, EPI, Diff, Asset, SPF, BV 1000
Ax. DWI	7000	min		250	128	192	22/22	5	0	1		SE, EPI, Diff, Asset, SPF, BV 2000
Ax.T2 FLAIR	9500	132	36	83.33	288	288	22/22	5	0	1.5	2375	FC, TRF, Propeller
Ax SWI	5000	Min	90 FA		192	320	22/22	2.4	0	4		EPI, FC, Freg R-1
Post GAD												
Ax Perfusion	2000	Min	FA60		96	128	22/22	7	0	1		GRE, MPh, EPI, 1 shot, Ramp Sampling On, 40 Locs/slice, Interleave

Quick protocol is used to demonstrate stroke/blood – in minimal scan time.
Use new 3D SWAN (susceptibility weighted imaging) when available for best visualization of blood.
Reformat with minimum rendering.
Perform perfusion when indicated. Post process as directed by radiologist.

Table 1-22   Site Protocol: Quick Stroke

Sequence 1.5	TR	TE	ETL/ FA	Band-width	F Matrix	Ph Matrix	FOV	Slice Thick	Inter-Space	NEX	TI	Pulse Sequence Options
Post GAD												

Table 1-22 Site Protocol: Quick Stroke—*cont'd*

Sequence 3T	TR	TE	ETL/FA	Band-width	F Matrix	Ph Matrix	FOV	Slice Thick	Inter-space	NEX	TI	Pulse Sequence Options
Post GAD												

Table 1-23 Brain–"Grab Bag"

Sequence 1.5	TR	TE	ETL/ FA	Band-width	F Matrix	Ph Matrix	FOV	Slice Thick	Inter-space	NEX	TI	Pulse Sequence Options
BRAVO	Mach	Min	FA 20	15.63	256	256	24/.75	1.4	124 locs	1	450	3DSPGR, lrP
T2 Cube	3000		100	62.50	288	288	24/24	1.4	116 locs	1		ZIP 2, ZIP 512, ARC
Flair Cube	6000		160	31.25	224	224	24/.90	1.4	116 locs	1	1850	ZIP 2, ZIP 512, IRP, ARC
Ax 3D Enhanced MRA	Min	Min	10 FA	20.83	320	256	22/22	1.4	110 locs	1		VAS PC, ASSET, ZIP 2, VENC 30-60, 19 Projections
Sag Enhanced MRV	Min	Min	10 FA	20.83	320	256	24/24	1.4	110 locs	1		ASSET, ZIP 2, VENC 15-20, 19 Projections
SWAN	78.3	50	15 FA	41.67	288	224	22/2	3	50 loc	1		Fast, FCn Zip 2, Asset
T1 STIR	1800	20		31.25	256	192	22.75	5	0	2	750	FC, Strong T1 contrast
Ax Perfusion	2000	27	FA60	31.25	128	128	24/24	10	40 locs/ slab	1		GRE, MPh, EPI, 1 shot, Ramp Sampling On, 40 Locs/slice, Interleave

Table 1-23	Brain–"Grab Bag" —cont'd											
Sequence 3T	TR	TE	ETL/ FA	Band-width	F Matrix	Ph Matrix	FOV	Slice Thick	Inter-space	NEX	TI	Pulse Sequence Options
BRAVO	Mach	Min	FA 12	31.25	320	320	24/.75	1.2	124 locs/ slice	1	400	3DSPGR, IrP
T2 Cube	3000		100	62.5	288	288	24	1.2		1		EDR, ZIP2, ZIP 512
Flair Cube	6000		140	31.25	224	224	24	1.2		1		EDR ZIP 512, ZIP2
Ax 3D Enhanced MRA	Min	Min	8FA	31.25	384	256	22/.90	1.2				VAS PC, ASSET, ZIP 2, VENC 30-60, 19 Projections
Sag Enhanced MRV	Min	Min	10 FA	20.83	320	256	24/24	1.4	110 locs	1		ASSET, ZIP 2, VENC 15-20, 19 Projections
Swan 3D	min	26	15	62.5	320	224	22	3.0	60 loc/ slab			Zip 2 FC and asset
Ax Perfusion	2000	Min	FA 60	–	96	128	22/22	7	40 locs/ slab	1		GRE, MPh, EPI, 1 shot, Ramp Sampling On, 40 Locs/slice, Interleave

Table 1-24 Site Protocol: Brain–"Grab Bag"

Sequence 1.5	TR	TE	ETL/FA	Band-width	F Matrix	Ph Matrix	FOV	Slice Thick	Inter-space	NEX	TI	Pulse Sequence Options
Post GAD												

Sequence 3T	TR	TE	ETL/FA	Band-width	F Matrix	Ph Matrix	FOV	Slice Thick	Inter-space	NEX	TI	Pulse Sequence Options
Post GAD												

Table 1-24 Site Protocol: Brain–"Grab Bag" —cont'd

fMRI—FUNCTIONAL MRI

Diffusion-Weighted Imaging

Diffusion-weighted imaging (DWI) is an echo planar imaging (EPI) sequence that detects random motion, or diffusion, of water molecules. This is done by adding two gradients to a spin-echo pulse sequence; the first dephases the water molecules and the second rephases them, and so recovers the signal lost during the first gradient. When water molecules move during the time between the gradients, the signal is not recovered, so tissues or fluid with higher water diffusion rates show more signal loss. The most common use for DWI is the diagnosis of acute stroke, In acute stroke there is "restricted diffusion" in the cytotoxic edema of the brain infarct so that water molecules move less than in normal brain tissue, show less signal loss, and appear as high-signal "bright" areas on DWI. This change occurs within minutes of the onset of ischemic stroke and is the most sensitive and specific way to diagnose brain infarction. DWI also shows high signal with restricted diffusion in TIA, demyelinating disease, bacterial abscess, and densely cellular neoplasms such as lymphoma.

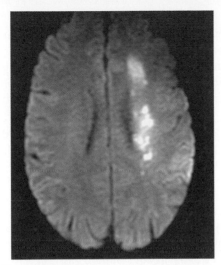

Figure 1-61 The diffusion-weighted image (DWI) shows abnormal high signal in the deep left frontal lobe, indicating an acute ischemic infarct. The "b" value is the shorthand term for a complex formula that indicates the strength of the diffusion gradients used to acquire this image. A value of b=1000 is the most common setting used for acute stroke detection.

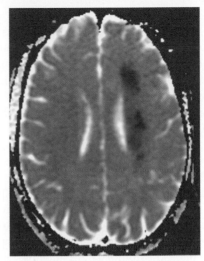

Figure 1-62 The apparent diffusion coefficient (ADC) map is a calculated map of the water diffusion rates in tissue. This ADC map shows the region of the acute infarct as low signal, corresponding to the high signal on DWI, and indicates that rate of water movement in the acute infarct is low or "restricted" in the cytotoxic edema of the acute infarct.

Diffusion Tensor Imaging

Diffusion tensor imaging (DTI) is a special application of the DWI sequence which enables diffusion to be measured in multiple directions (6 or more). The rate of diffusion in these multiple directions is then processed mathematically to derive an overall direction within each imaging voxel, called a "tensor." This is used to construct the shape of water diffusion in the voxel in a range from spherical (the same rate of diffusion in all directions) to linear (diffusion only along a single direction). Diffusion in most voxels in tissue produces the shape of a distorted sphere, called an ellipsoid, which in the brain is almost spherical in highly cellular gray matter and more elongated in white matter (along the direction of the white matter axons). The degree of this distortion from a sphere is summarized numerically as a "fractional anisotropy" (FA) value between 0.0 (spherical or "isotropic" diffusion) and 1.0 (maximally elongated or "anisotropic" diffusion) so that gray matter has low FA values around 0.1 and white matter has higher FA values around 0.5.

This information can then be used to generate white matter tract maps, also called "tractography," by mathematically linking the elongated ellipsoids of adjacent voxels together to form lines that represent white matter "fibers" and bundles of these fibers that represent white matter "tracts." The mathematical rules for linking ellipsoids from one voxel to the next can be adjusted to include or exclude some white matter or change the size and direction of tracts, so these "tract maps" should be viewed only as estimates of the true white matter tracts. They are also only mathematical estimates of white matter structure and do not indicate whether the white matter is functioning normally.

Also keep in mind that increased water from edema around white matter tracts can create more spherical diffusion around them (reducing the FA) and so prevent linking of voxels and "hide" normal white matter running through the edema. For example, the absence of white matter tracts in the edema around a brain tumor does not mean that the surgeon can safely remove that tissue because it may contain "hidden," normal white matter fibers. On the other hand, diseases of the white matter often reduce the diffusion along the direction of the axons (reducing the FA) and result in loss of tract mapping. This change can be seen as reduced signal on FA maps and tract maps and is used to evaluate patients with demyelinating disease such as multiple sclerosis or injury to white matter tracts from trauma or stroke. DTI tractography is also being used to study the abnormal organization of white matter tracts, or "abnormal wiring" in the brain with disorders such as epilepsy, autism, or schizophrenia.

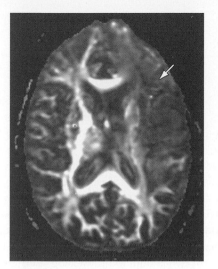

Figure 1-63 This diffusion tensor "fractional anisotropy" (FA) map shows reduced signal in the left-sided brain tumor and surrounding edema, indicating more spherical diffusion (low FA). There is apparent absence of the normal white matter tracts in this region (*arrow*), which are seen as curvilinear high-signal structures in the opposite hemisphere. This may mean either that these white matter tracts are abnormal from disease (tumor infiltration) or normal and simply "hidden" by the effect of surrounding edema. Because these tract maps only reflect structure and do not indicate function, the surgeon needs to approach these areas cautiously to avoid damage to normally functioning white matter tracts.

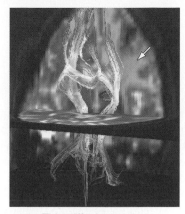

Figure 1-64 This diffusion tensor "tractography map" shows the estimated course of white matter fibers and tracts in color based on mathematical criteria for linking diffusion tensor ellipsoids from one voxel to the next. Higher FA and similar diffusion tensor direction is needed to produce a link and create a "fiber" mathematically. The region of reduced mapping in the left frontal lobe around the brain tumor and in the region of edema is a direct effect of the reduced FA in this region (*arrow*). As in the FA map, this may mean either that these white matter tracts are abnormal from disease (tumor infiltration) or normal and simply "hidden" by the effect of surrounding edema.

Perfusion-Weighted Imaging

Perfusion-weighted imaging (PWI) is also called dynamic susceptibility contrast (DSC) imaging and is based on the transient effect of a bolus of intravascular, paramagnetic gadolinium contrast passing through brain tissue. The high concentration of the gadolinium bolus in the arteries, capillaries, and veins creates a dynamic, local change in magnetic susceptibility around the vessels, resulting in low signal on T2* EPI gradient echo images (spin dephasing by the local gradients around the vessels). This produces a "negative contrast" downward-pointing signal curve in each voxel as the bolus passes through the tissue. This curve can then be analyzed mathematically to produce maps of the components of tissue perfusion including cerebral blood flow (CBF), cerebral blood volume (CBV), and mean transit time (MTT). They key components of this "first pass" bolus curve are the baseline signal before the bolus arrives (1), the steep "wash-in" downward slope as the bolus arrives (2), the negative "peak" at the maximum bolus concentration (3), and the "wash-out" upward slope as the bolus leaves the tissue (4) (see lower, normal curve in Figure 1-65).

Hemodynamic analysis of the curve is commonly based on the "central volume principle" relationship between CBF, CBV, and MTT (CBF=CBV/MTT), where CBV is calculated as the area under the bolus curve, measured from the extended pre-bolus baseline, and the MTT is estimated as the width of the curve at the half maximum point of the bolus curve. More direct measurements of the curve components are also used to simplify processing, such as the steepness of the wash-in slope for CBF and the time-to-peak (TTP) of the curve as a substitute for MTT. Because there are many source of uncertainty in these measurements with MRI, absolute quantitation of hemodynamic parameters is difficult and these values are usually expressed as "relative" measures between different brain regions, typically abbreviated as rCBF, rCBV, rMTT, and rTTP. Software for processing these curves into hemodynamic maps is available from all commercial MRI vendors. The common clinical applications of this information include mapping of the region of prolonged rMTT and reduced rCBV and rCBF with cerebrovascular stenosis or cerebral ischemia with stroke and estimation of the rCBV in primary brain tumor as an indicator of the degree of malignancy (grade). Another MRI method of measuring cerebral blood flow, called arterial spin labeling (ASL), can be done without the use of a gadolinium contrast injection but is technically more challenging and less widely available. A detailed description of this method is beyond the scope of this article.

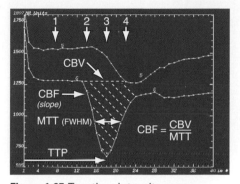

Figure 1-65 Two time-intensity curves during the passage of a gadolinium bolus through brain tissue. The lower curve represents normal perfusion with a steep, narrow perfusion curve indicating normal cerebral blood flow (CBF), cerebral blood volume (CBV), mean transit time (MTT), and time-to-peak (TTP). The upper curve represents ischemic tissue with reduced CBF, reduced CBV, prolonged MTT, and delayed TTP

The DWI image (1-66) shows abnormal high signal in the right frontal and right parietal lobes. The corresponding ADC map (1-68) shows the lowest signal in the right frontal lesion (70% below the comparable normal contralateral region), indicating an acute infarct with severe "diffusion restriction." The parietal lesion shows minimal ADC reduction of 30%, indicating a subacute infarct with partial reversal of diffusion restriction, called "pseudonormalization." The perfusion maps show abnormally increased TTP (1-67, left image), reduced CBF (1-69) and reduced CBV (1-70) in the acute right frontal infarct with normal values in the right parietal lesion, typical of "reflow" to a subacute infarct.

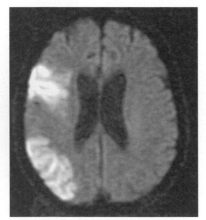

Figure 1-66

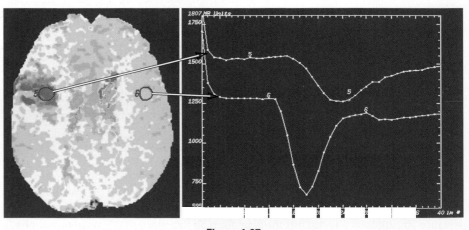

Figure 1-67

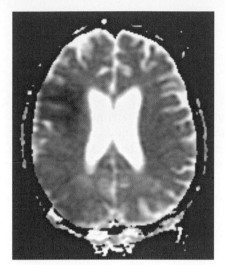

Figure 1-68

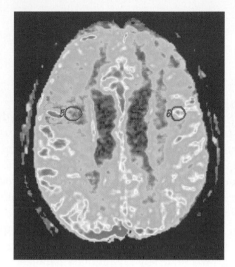

Figure 1-69

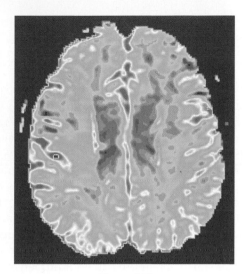

Figure 1-70

MR Spectroscopy

MR Spectroscopy (MRS) is a method that displays proton signals from certain metabolites in tissue by looking at the unique radio-frequency of specific molecules. These molecules are present in very small concentrations compared with water in tissue so the molecular signals are not visible on standard MR images. Specialized pulse sequences are used to suppress the large water signal to see these small signals. Specialized techniques are also used to "shim" the magnetic field and improve homogeneity within the acquired volume of interest (voxel) to maximize sensitivity to the low concentrations of these molecules. The result of the MRS acquisition are displayed graphically as a spectrum of peaks whose height and width are proportional to the concentration of the specific molecule in the tissue. The separation of peaks in this graphical display is based on the difference in magnetic resonance frequency between the molecules and is shown on a relative scale of parts per million (ppm) so that results from different magnetic field strengths can be compared. MRS can be acquired from a signal voxel in which all of the signal is averaged into one spectrum, giving the maximum signal-to-noise ratio (SNR) or from multiple voxels subdividing the acquisition volume, which gives separate spectra from smaller, more focused regions (e.g. separate spectra from tumor and normal brain) but with lower SNR. Because precise quantitation of metabolites with MRS is difficult in living tissue, clinical applications rely on the pattern of peak heights of the most common metabolites. For example, many pathologic processes in the brain reduce the concentration of a metabolite that is specific to neurons, N-acetylaspartate (NAA), but do not change the high-energy phosphate storage molecule Creatine (Cr) so changes in NAA are usually expressed as the ratio of NAA to Creatine (NAA/Cr). Other ratios are also used to help characterize brain lesions such as Choline (Cho) relative to Cr (Cho/Cr). High-grade brain tumors can show both elevated Cho/Cr and reduced NAA/Cr (Figure 1-71). The following metabolites are commonly visualized when performing MRS of the brain (annotated in parts per million, PPM):

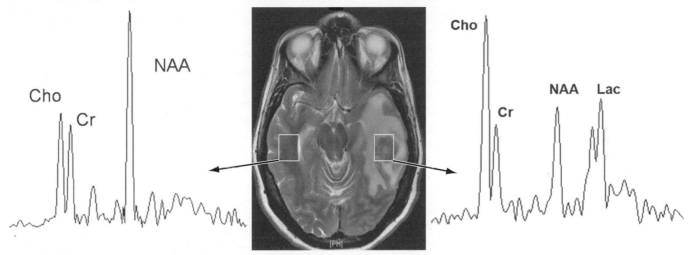

Figure 1-71 Normal brain MRS with normal metabolite rations of Cho/Cr (1.2) and NAA/Cr (2.4) and normal glucose energy metabolism with no lactate

Abnormal brain tumor MRS with abnormal metabolite ratios of elevated Cho/Cr (2.2) and reduced NAA (1.3) and abnormal glucose energy metabolism with a large

lactate peak (with a characteristic split "doublet" peak)

KEY: MRS, magnetic resonance spectroscopy.

Choline (Cho): A metabolite from cellular membranes, which may be elevated during membrane production (e.g. tumor) or membrane destruction (e.g., demyelination). Peak occurs at 3.2 ppm.

Creatine (Cr): A cellular energy storage molecule for high-energy phosphates, which is relatively stable across many conditions and pathologies (and often used as the reference peak for other metabolites). Peak occurs at 3.03 ppm.

- Myo-inositol (mI): Hormone-sensitive neuron-reception mechanisms. Increased in Alzheimer disease and decreased in hepatic encephalopathy. Peak occurs at 3.56 ppm
- When performing a MRS for brain tumor, the CHO and NAA peaks are reversed in amplitude when a tumor is present. Normally the CHO peak is higher than the NAA peak, but in tumor the NAA is higher and the CHO is reduced.

Functional MRI

Functional MRI (fMRI) is usually performed using the Blood Oxygen Level Dependent (BOLD) method, which maps the increase in signal in the brain with local increases in blood flow and blood oxygen that occur with neuronal "activation" when a person is performing a task. A T2* sequence is used to detect this local hemodynamic response (change in blood flow) because it is sensitive to microscopic magnetic susceptibility changes around blood vessels. As the blood oxygen levels change, there is a change in the ratio of oxyhemoglobin (red blood cell hemoglobin saturated with oxygen) to deoxyhemoglobin (hemoglobin without oxygen, after oxygen has been released to the tissue). Oxyhemoglobin is magnetically neutral and does not produce magnetic susceptibility changes around blood vessels. Deoxyhemoglobin is paramagnetic and higher concentrations in blood produce magnetic susceptibility gradients at the blood vessel wall, resulting in low signal on T2* images. Normal "resting" brain tissue has a relatively high level of deoxyhemoglobin and so appears dark. "Activated" brain stimulates increased local blood flow, which brings in more oxyhemoglobin and decreases deoxyhemoglobin, resulting in reduced magnetic susceptibility gradients around blood vessels and increased local signal on T2* images. This local signal increase is often referred to as the BOLD "activation" on fMRI studies.

Images of local signal increases during BOLD fMRI are generated by rapidly acquiring echo-planar (EPI) T2* images while the subject performs a task, then comparing the higher signal during the task to the lower signal during a rest period. The most common fMRI "task paradigm" is a "block" design, which alternates task activity with rest periods between the tasks. The rapid sequence of T2* images is then processed using "correlation analysis" to look through voxels in the entire brain for regions that show a similar timing pattern (correlation) between the local signal increases and the task activity, compared with the lower signal during the rest periods. More repetitions of the task during the fMRI acquisition increase the confidence level of this analysis. These results are then displayed as a map with color coding to show the confidence level of the correlation (typically higher confidence levels in red on a rainbow color scale). A display of the signal curve during the repeated tasks may also be used for a visual evaluation of the quality of the correlation. There are several commercially available fMRI activation systems that include a range of paradigm designs, audio-visual stimulation technology, and sophisticated data analysis. Depending on the purpose of the study, subjects may perform motor-sensory tasks (e.g., finger tapping), language tasks (e.g., picture naming or word generation), cognitive tasks, memory tasks, or may passively view movies, hear sounds or smell odors. The variety of possible tasks and stimuli make fMRI a very powerful technique for clinical evaluation and scientific research into brain function.

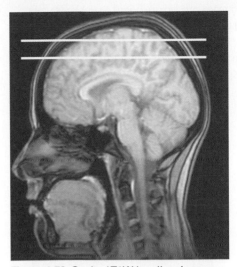

Figure 1-72 Sagittal T1W localizer image shows the location of the axial fMRI images acquired through the primary motor and sensory cortex during a motor-sensory activation task

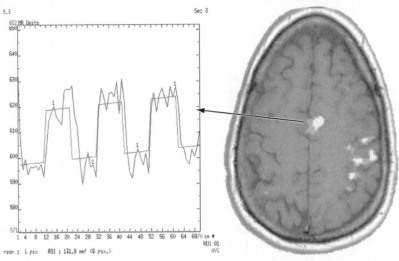

Figure 1-73 Left, BOLD signal curve from an activation region over the course of a "block" design task paradigm visually demonstrates the strong correlation between activation and task. **Right**, Axial anatomic image with overlaid "activation map" showing voxels with the highest correlation between BOLD signal and the task paradigm during right-hand finger tapping.

SOFT TISSUE NECK

Acquire three-plane pilot per site specifications for soft tissue neck.

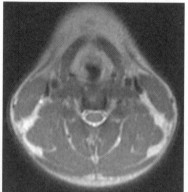

Figure 1-74 Axial image of the neck

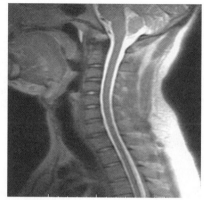

Figure 1-75 Sagittal image of the neck

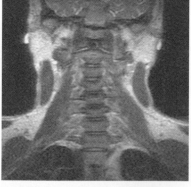

Figure 1-76 Coronal image of the neck

COIL: Multi-channel neurovascular

POSITION: Supine, head first; place cushion under knees or multi-channel head spine coil

LANDMARK: Sternal notch

IMMOBILIZATION: Place cushions around the head; tape with gauze across the forehead. Have the patient minimize swallowing during the scanning acquisition to avoid artifacts across the image.

Make sure to scan inferiorly to below the aortic arch when vocal cord paralysis is suspected.

The vagus nerve that controls the vocal cords extends below the aortic arch.

> **TIP:** Saline bags or fat pads placed bilateral to the neck will help to improve fat saturation. If T2 fat sat is not effective, inversion recovery can be used. When it is available, use the IDEAL sequence (fat/water separation) for uniform fat suppression.

Acquisition of Coronal Images of the Neck

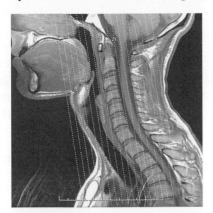

Figure 1-77 Sagittal image of the neck with coronal locations

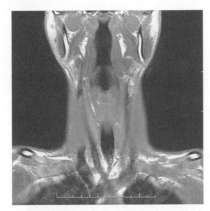

Figure 1-78 Coronal image of the neck

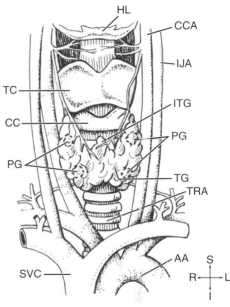

Figure 1-79 Coronal anatomy of the neck

SLICE ACQUISITION: Anterior to posterior

SLICE ALIGNMENT: Parallel to the vertebral bodies

ANATOMIC COVERAGE: Anterior from hyoid bone to the spinous process, superior from the hard palate to the arch of the aorta

KEY: **AA**, aortic arch; **CC**, cricoid cartilage; **CCA**, common carotid artery; **HL**, hyoid bone; **IJA**, internal jugular vein; **ITG**, isthmus of thyroid gland; **PG**, parathyroid glands; **SVC**, superior vena cava; **TC**, thyroid cartilage; **TG**, thyroid gland; **TRA**, trachea.

Acquisition of Axial Images of the Neck

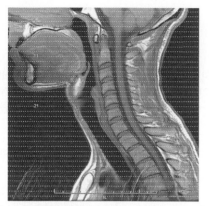

Figure 1-80 Sagittal image of the neck with axial locations

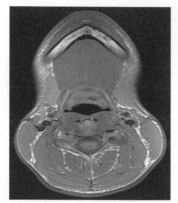

Figure 1-81 Axial image of the neck at level of C4

Figure 1-82 Axial anatomy of the neck at level of C4

SLICE ACQUISITION: Superior to inferior

SLICE ALIGNMENT: Parallel to hard palate.

ANATOMIC COVERAGE: For vocal cord paralysis scan from hard palate to arch of the aorta. For neck mass scan from hard palate to sternal notch.

KEY: **ECA,** external carotid artery; **EJV,** external jugular vein; **ICA,** internal carotid artery; **IJV,** internal jugular vein; **M,** mandible; **O,** oropharynx; **PG,** parotid gland; **SC,** spinal cord; **SG,** submandibular gland; **SM,** sternocleidomastoid muscle; **T,** tongue.

Table 1-25 Soft Tissue Neck

Sequence 1.5	TR	TE	ETL or FA	Band-width	F Matrix	Ph Matrix	FOV	Slice Thick	Inter-space	NEX	TI	Pulse Sequence Options
Cor STIR FSE	4000	68	17	41.67	384	224	26/26	5	.5	3	110	FC, seq
Ax T1 FSE	600	Min	4	41.67	320	224	24/24	5	1.5	2		Sat S-I, NPW
Ax T2 FSE	3300	110	27	41.67	256	224	24/24	5	1.5	3		FC, NPW
Post GAD												
Ax 3D SPGR FS	40	Min	40FA	15.63	224	224	24/.75	4	0	2		FS, FC, ZIP 512
Sag 3D FSPGR FS		In phase	40FA	62.50	256	256	24/24	4	40 slab	1.5		Sat S-I, Fat, NPW, ZIP 512

(Continued)

Table 1-25 Soft Tissue Neck—*cont'd*

Sequence 3T	TR	TE	ETL or FA	Band-width	F Matrix	Ph Matrix	FOV	Slice Thick	Inter-space	NEX	TI	Pulse Sequence Options
Cor STIR	4500	68	31	50	320	224	26/26	5	.5	3	170	FC, Seq
Ax. T1	1100	Min	4	50	320	224	24/24	5	1	2		Sat S-I, NPW
Ax. T2	4600	85	17	52.50	288	224	24/24	5	1	2		FC, NPW
Post GAD												
Ax .3D FSPGR IR PREP		Min	20FA	31.25	256	192	24	4	70 loc/slab	1	450	IR PREP, FC, ZIP 512, ZIP 2
Sag .3D FSPGR IR PREP		Min	20FA	31.25	256	192	26	4	70 loc/slab	1	450	3D FSPGR, IR PREP, FC, ZIP 512, ZIP 2

T1 FSE ETL 4 or lower.

When Coronal SPGR C+ acquisition is requested by a radiologist, use sagittal acquisition and change it into a coronal plane.

Use IDEAL sequence in the coronal plane when available.

TRF (Tailor Radio-Frequency) should be used with all FSE sequence to increase # of slices per TR.

Table 1-26 Site Protocol: Soft Tissue Neck

Sequence 1.5	TR	TE	ETL or FA	Band-width	F Matrix	Ph Matrix	FOV	Slice Thick	Inter-space	NEX	TI	Pulse Sequence Options
Post GAD												

(Continued)

Table 1-26 Site Protocol: Soft Tissue Neck—*cont'd*

Sequence 3T	TR	TE	ETL or FA	Band-width	F Matrix	Ph Matrix	FOV	Slice Thick	Inter-space	NEX	TI	Pulse Sequence Options
Post GAD												

MAGNETIC RESONANCE ANGIOGRAPHY OF CAROTID ARTERIES AND CAROTID BIFURCATION

Acquire three-plane pilot per site specifications.

Acquisition of Coronal PC Localizer

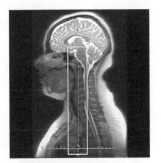

Figure 1-83 Sagittal image of the neck with coronal locations for vessels

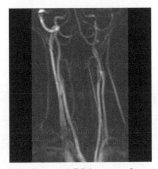

Figure 1-84 Coronal PC image of vessels

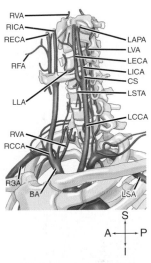

Figure 1-85 Coronal anatomy of vessels

KEY: BA, brachiocephalic artery; **CS**, carotid sinus; **LCCA**, left common carotid artery; **LECA**, left external carotid artery; **LICA**, left internal carotid artery; **LSA**, left subclavian artery; **LVA**, left vertebral artery; **RCCA**, right common carotid artery; **RECA**, right external carotid artery; **RFA**, right facial artery; **RICA**, right internal carotid artery; **RSA**, right subclavian artery; **RVA**, right vertebral artery.

COIL: Multi-channel neurovascular or multi-channel head coil
POSITION: Supine, head first with cushion under knees
LANDMARK: Mental protuberance (chin)
IMMOBILIZATION: Place cushions around the head, and tape with gauze across the forehead.

TIP: Ask the patient not to swallow during the scanning acquisition to avoid an artifact across the bifurcation. A vendor-specific PC sequence most effectively localizes vessels.

Acquisition of Two-Dimensional TOF

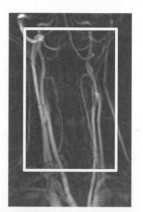

Figure 1-86 Coronal image of neck with axial locations for bilateral of carotid arteries

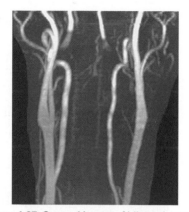

Figure 1-87 Coronal image of bilateral carotid arteries

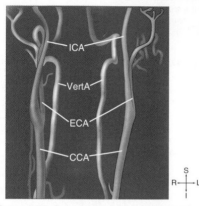

Figure 1-88 Coronal anatomy of bilateral carotid arteries

SLICE ACQUISITION: Inferior to superior
SLICE ALIGNMENT: Perpendicular to vessels
ANATOMIC COVERAGE: From superior subclavian arteries to the vertebral-basilar junction

KEY: **CCA**, common carotid artery; **ECA**, external carotid artery; **ICA**, internal carotid artery; **VertA**, vertebral artery.

TIP: Place a superior saturation band to eliminate venous flow. Images should be post processed to separate left and right carotid (GE IVId), for better visualization of anatomy.

Acquisition of Three-Dimensional TOF: Carotid Bifurcation

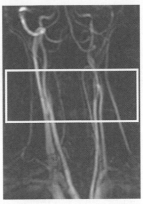

Figure 1-89 Coronal image with axial locs for carotid bifurcation

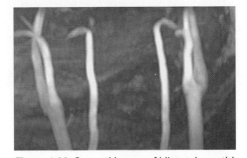

Figure 1-90 Coronal image of bilateral carotid bifurcation

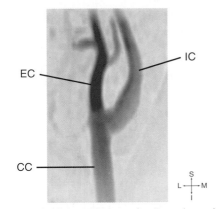

Figure 1-91 Coronal image of unilateral carotid bifurcation

KEY: **CC**, common carotid; **EC**, external carotid; **IC**, internal carotid.

SLICE ACQUISITION: Inferior to superior

SLICE ALIGNMENT: Perpendicular to vessels

ANATOMIC COVERAGE: Superior and inferior to the bifurcation

TIP: Place a superior saturation band (Sat S), to eliminate venous flow. Images should be post processed to separate left and right carotid for better visualization.

Table 1-27 MRA Carotids and Carotid Bifurcation

Sequence 1.5	TR	TE	ETL or FA	Band-width	F Matrix	Ph Matrix	FOV	Slice Thick	Interspace	NEX	TI	Pulse Sequence Options
COR 2D PC	33	Min	20FA	15.63	256	160	35/.75	60	0	4		VAS PC, Venc 50 cm/sec, FC, flow all direction
2DTOF	Min	Min	60 FA	20.83	320	192	22/.50	2.0	-.8	2		SPGR Vas TOF, Sat S, FC, seq
3DTOF	53	Min	20FA	15.63	288	192	22/.81	2	34 loc/slab	1		SPGR Vas TOF, Sat S and fat, MgT, Zip 512, Zip 2, Rmp Pulse I-S
OPT T1 FS	600	Min	3-4	31.25	256	224	22/22	5	0	2		Sat I, F
Post GAD												
Cor. 3D TRICKS		Min	FA30	31.25	256	192	28/.75	4	0 Locs 18	1		3D TRICKS, ZIP 512, ZIP 2, 18 scan locs, Temp Resol 3-4, Scan 15 times

Table 1-27 MRA Carotids and Carotid Bifurcation—*cont'd*

Sequence 3T	TR	TE	ETL or FA	Band-width	F Matrix	Ph Matrix	FOV	Slice Thick	Inter-space	NEX	TI	Pulse Sequence Options
COR 2D PC	30	Min	30FA	31.25	256	192	30/.75	30	0	4		VAS PC, Venc 40 cm/sec, FC, flow all direction
2DTOF	Min	Min	80FA	31.25	320	192	22/.50	2.0	-.8	2		SPGR Vas TOF, Sat S, FC, Seq
3DTOF	45	Min	45FA	15.63	288	192	22/.81	2	34 loc/slab	1		SPGR Vas TOF, Sat S and Fat, MgT, Zip 512, Zip 2, Rmp Pulse I-S
OPT T1 FS	600	Min	3-4	41.67	256	224	22/22	5	0	1		Sat I, F
Post GAD												
Cor. 3D TRICKS		Min	FA30	125	256	192	28/.75	4	0 Locs 18	1		3D TRICKS, ZIP 512, ZIP 2, 18 scan locs, Temp Resol 3-4, Scan 15 times

Use coronal PC loc to best visualize vessels.
Scan TOF bottom to top. Reformat left and right side separately.
OPT (optional) T1 FS should be included when indication is for dissection.
Time resolved imaging (TRICKS-GE) is obtained when contrast is indicated. Scan from the arch to COW (Circle of Willis).

Table 1-28   Site Protocol: MRA Carotids and Carotid Bifurcation

Sequence 1.5	TR	TE	ETL/FA	Band-width	F Matrix	Ph Matrix	FOV	Slice Thick	Inter-space	NEX	TI	Pulse Sequence Options
Post GAD												

Sequence 3T	TR	TE	ETL/FA	Band-width	F Matrix	Ph Matrix	FOV	Slice Thick	Inter-space	NEX	TI	Pulse Sequence Options
Post GAD												

Table 1-28 Site Protocol: Carotids and Carotid Bifurcation—*cont'd*

MRI of the Spine and Bony Pelvis

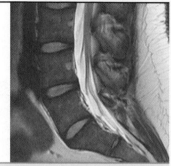

MRI OF THE SPINE AND BONY PELVIS—CONSIDERATIONS

- Refer to all safety-related parameters discussed in Chapter 1.
- As the SAR increases, the patient's body temperature will also increase. At 3 T make sure your estimated SAR is 2.5 or lower before scanning to keep the SAR at an acceptable rate. The SAR elevation can be compensated for by increasing the TR slightly. If this is not done correctly, the SAR will increase and the scanner will stop as a patient safety precaution. All 3-T systems have SAR monitors that should be referenced while scanning. This is not an issue at 1.5 T.
- An eight-channel or higher vendor-specific CTL coil is used primarily to image the spine. The CTL coil is divided into specific sections to correspond to segments of the vertebral column.
- All multichannel coils produce excessive signal adjacent to the coil. This can be compensated for by using vendor-specific options (e.g., GE uses SCIC or PURE to provide uniform signal intensity).
- Generally at 3 T, in the spine, T1 FLAIR is substituted for T1 spin-echo or fast spin echo to compensate for long T1 relaxation times at 3 T.
- T1 and T1 FLAIR imaging are best used to identify anatomic structure, whereas T2 and T2 FLAIR imaging provide detailed evidence of pathologic conditions.
- On T1 sequences, CSF produces dark or hypointense signal. T1 FLAIR uses an inversion pulse also to produce dark or hypointense signal.
- On T2 sequences, CSF produces bright or hyperintense signal. T2 FLAIR uses an inversion pulse to produce dark or hypointense CSF signal; all other fluid appears bright.
- Superior and inferior saturation bands help to compensate for CSF and vascular pulsation, whereas anterior saturation bands can help compensate for breathing, swallowing, and peristalsis. Saturation bands can be used on all pulse sequences.
- Fat saturation options and terminology are vendor specific. For GE systems, use "fat classic" for fat saturation with enhanced anatomic detail.
- When trauma, infection, or tumor is suspected, T2 fat saturation or short T1 inversion recovery images should be performed to enhance abnormal fluid or pathology.
- Flow compensation or gradient nulling should be used on T2 images to help compensate for CSF flow and vascular motion. Flow compensation should never be used on T1 precontrast because it causes vessels to appear bright and to mimic pathologic conditions. It is often used post gadolinium on T1 sequences to compensate for flow artifacts.

ROUTINE CERVICAL SPINE

Acquire three-plane pilot per site specifications.

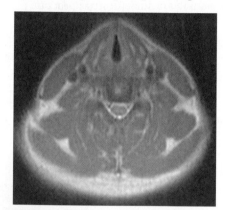

Figure 2-1 Axial image of the cervical spine

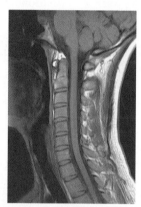

Figure 2-2 Sagittal image of the cervical spine

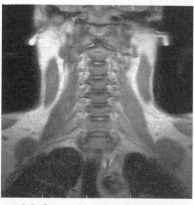

Figure 2-3 Coronal image of the cervical spine

COIL: Multi-channel coil
POSITION: Supine, head first, cushion under knees
LANDMARK: Hyoid bone, thyroid cartilage
IMMOBILIZATION: Prevent the body from touching the sides of the magnet by using sponges or sheets.

Acquisition of Sagittal Images of the Cervical Spine

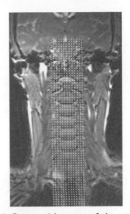

Figure 2-4 Coronal image of the cervical spine with sagittal locations

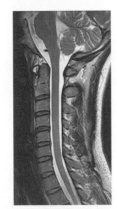

Figure 2-5 Sagittal image of the cervical spine with anterior saturation band

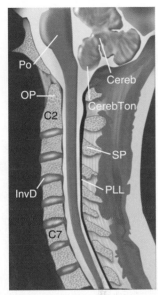

Figure 2-6 Sagittal anatomy of the cervical spine

SLICE ACQUISITION: Left to right
SLICE ALIGNMENT: Parallel to spinal cord and margins of vertebral bodies
ANATOMIC COVERAGE: Cerebellum to thoracic 1, left to right margins of vertebral bodies

TIP: "Anterior" saturation band in the field of view will help to compensate for patient swallowing.

KEY: **Cereb**, cerebellum; **CerebTon**, cerebral tonsil; **InvD**, intervertebral disk; **OP**, odontoid process; **Po**, pons; **PLL**, poster longitudinal ligament; **SP**, spinous process.

Acquisition of Axial Images of the Cervical Spine

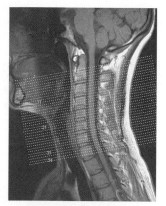

Figure 2-7 Sagittal image with axial locations and anterior saturation band

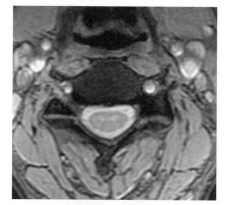

Figure 2-8 Axial image of the cervical spine

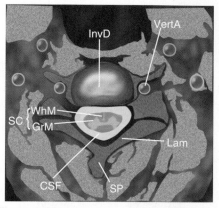

Figure 2-9 Axial anatomy of the cervical spine

SLICE ACQUISITION: Superior to inferior
SLICE ALIGNMENT: Parallel to the intervertebral joint spaces
ANATOMIC COVERAGE: C2 through T1

KEY: **CSF**, cerebral spinal fluid; **GrM**, gray matter; **InvD**, intervertebral disk; **Lam**, lamina; **SC**, spinal cord; **SP**, spinous process; **VertA**, vertebral artery; **WhM**, white matter.

Table 2-1 Routine Cervical Spine

Sequence 1.5	TR	TE	ETL or FA	Band-width	F Matrix	Ph Matrix	FOV	Slice Thick	Inter-space	NEX	TI	Pulse Sequence Options
Sag. T2 FSE	3400	102	14	41.67	320	224	24/24	3	1	4		Sat A, S-I, FC, NPW, SPF
Sag. T1 FSE	450	14	4	35.71	256	224	24/24	3	1	4		Sat A, NPW, SPF
Sag STIR	2888	60	10	41.67	256	224	24/24	3	0	3	110	FSE-IR, Sat A, S-I, FC, Seq
Ax 3D Cosmic	—	—	FA 40	50	320	288	18	2.8	0	1		Cosmic, Sat S, I, Zip 2
Ax.T2 FRFSE	3000	110	21	31.25	256	224	20/20	4	0	4		Sat A, FC, NPW
Post GAD												
Ax.T1 FSE	625	Min	3	41.67	256	224	20/20	4	0	2		Sat F, A, NPW
Sag. T1 FS FSE	450	14	4	35.71	256	224	24/24	3	1	4		Sat A, NPW

(Continued)

| Table 2-1 | Routine Cervical Spine—*cont'd* |

Sequence 3T	TR	TE	ETL or FA	Band-width	F Matrix	Ph Matrix	FOV	Slice Thick	Inter-space	NEX	TI	Pulse Sequence Options
Sag. T2 FRFSE	4000	110	21	41.67	416	224	24/24	3	.5	4		Sat A, S-I, FC, NPW
Sag.T1 Flair	3000	22	8	41.67	448	224	24/24	4	1	2	Auto	Sat S-I, A, seq, NPW
Sag STIR	4550	42	10	41.67	288	192	24/24	3	0	3	200	FSE-IR, Sat A, S-I, FC, Seq
Ax 2D Merge	940	—	FA 40	41.67	288	192	18/18	3	.3	2		Merge, FC, NPW
Ax.T2 FRFSE	3200	85	17	50	288	224	18/18	4	0	4		Sat A, FC, NPW
Post GAD												
Ax.T1 FSE	1100	Min	4	50	256	224	18/18	4	0	2		Sat A, NPW
Sag.T1 FLAIR FS	3000	22	8	41.67	448	224	24/24	4	1	2	Auto	Sat S-I, A, Seq, NPW

Add pre contrast T1 Ax when Gadolinium is administrated.
T1 FS ETL 4 of lower.
Add a coronal T2 when patient has scoliosis or tethered cord.
TRF (Tailor Radio-Frequency) should be used with all FSE sequence to increase # of slices per TR.
SPF (Swap phase and frequency) is used to reduce CSF artifacts.
Use NPW when possibility of anatomy wrapping (No Phase Wrap).
Use IDEAL when available (see grab bag).

Table 2-2 Site Protocol Cervical Spine

Sequence 1.5	TR	TE	ETL or FA	Band-width	F Matrix	Ph Matrix	FOV	Slice Thick	Inter-space	NEX	TI	Pulse Sequence Options
Post GAD												

(Continued)

Table 2-2   Site Protocol Cervical Spine—*cont'd*

Sequence 3T	TR	TE	ETL or FA	Band-width	F Matrix	Ph Matrix	FOV	Slice Thick	Inter-space	NEX	TI	Pulse Sequence Options
Post GAD												

CERVICAL SPINE FOR MULTIPLE SCLEROSIS

Table 2-3   Cervical Spine for Multiple Sclerosis

Sequence 1.5	TR	TE	ETL or FA	Band-width	F Matrix	Ph Matrix	FOV	Slice Thick	Inter-space	NEX	TI	Pulse Sequence Options
Sag. T2 FRFSE	3400	102	14	41.67	320	224	24/24	3	0	4		Sat A, S-I, FC, SPF
Sag STIR	2888	60	10	41.67	256	224	24/24	3	0	3	110	FSE-IR, Sat A, S-I, FC, seq
Sag. T1 FSE	450	14	4	35.71	256	224	24/24	3	1	4		Sat A, S-I
Ax.T2 FRFSE	3300	110	27	35.71	256	224	20/.75	4	0	3		Sat A, S-I, FC, Zip 512
Ax.T1 FSE	625	Min	3	41.67	256	224	20/20	4	0	2		Sat A, S-I
Post GAD												
Ax.T1 FSE	625	Min	3	41.67	256	224	20/20	4	0	2		Sat F, A, S-I
Sag. T1 FS FSE	450	14	4	35.71	256	224	24/24	3	1	4		Sat A, S-I, Fat, SPF

(Continued)

Table 2-3												Cervical Spine for Multiple Sclerosis—*cont'd*
Sequence 3T	TR	TE	ETL or FA	Band-width	F Matrix	Ph Matrix	FOV	Slice Thick	Inter-space	NEX	TI	Pulse Sequence Options
Sag. T2 FRFSE	4000	110	21	41.67	416	224	24/24	3	.5	4		Sat A, S-I, FC, SPF
Sag STIR	4550	42	10	41.67	288	192	24/24	3	0	3	200	FSE-IR, Sat A, S-I, FC, seq
Sag.T1 Flair	3000	22	8	41.67	448	224	24/24	4	1	2	Auto	Sat S-I, A, seq, SPF
Ax.T2 FRFSE	3200	85	17	50	288	224	18/18	4	0	4		Sat A, FC
Ax.T1 FSE	1100	Min	4	50	256	224	18/18	4	0	2		Sat A
Post GAD												
Ax.T1 FSE	1100	Min	4	50	256	224	18/18	4	0	2		Sat A
Sag.T1 Flair FS	3000	22	8	41.67	448	224	24/24	4	1	2	Auto	Sat S-I, A, TRF, seq, SPF

T1 FSE ETL 4 of lower.
TRF (Tailor Radio-Frequency) should be used with all FSE sequences to increase # of slices per TR.
SPF (Swap phase and frequency) is used to reduce CSF artifacts.
Use NPW when possibility of anatomy wrapping (No Phase Wrap).
Use IDEAL when available (see grab bag).

Table 2-4 Site Protocol: Multiple Sclerosis

Sequence 1.5	TR	TE	ETL or FA	Band-width	F Matrix	Ph Matrix	FOV	Slice Thick	Inter-space	NEX	TI	Pulse Sequence Options
Post GAD												

(Continued)

Table 2-4	Site Protocol: Multiple Sclerosis—*cont'd*											
Sequence 3T	TR	TE	ETL or FA	Band-width	F Matrix	Ph Matrix	FOV	Slice Thick	Inter-space	NEX	TI	Pulse Sequence Options
Post GAD												

ROUTINE THORACIC SPINE

For anatomic reference, acquire an extended field of view pilot from the base of the brain through the thoracic spine.

This allows for accurate identification of vertebral levels.

Acquire three-plane pilot per site specifications.

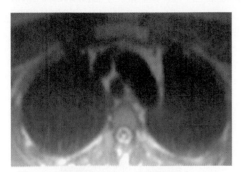

Figure 2-10 Axial image of thoracic spine

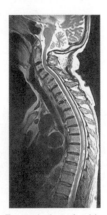

Figure 2-11 Extended sagittal image of thoracic spine (48 FOV)

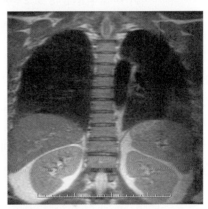

Figure 2-12 Coronal image of thoracic spine

COIL: Multi-channel or HNS2-3-4

POSITION: Supine, head first, cushion under knees

LANDMARK: Midsternum, 2 to 3 inches superior to xiphoid

IMMOBILIZATION: Prevent the body from touching the sides of the magnet with sponges or sheets. Velcro bands may be used across the torso.

TIP: If the patient is severely kyphotic, place cushions under the buttocks and thighs. If the patient has scoliosis, a detailed coronal image (48 FOV) will assist in plotting the sagittal sequences.

Acquisition of Sagittal Image

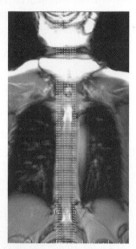

Figure 2-13 Coronal image of thoracic spine with sagittal locs

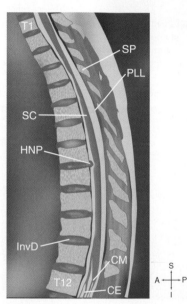

Figure 2-14 Sagittal image of the thoracic spine

Figure 2-15 Sagittal anatomy of the thoracic spine

SLICE ACQUISITION: Left to right

SLICE ALIGNMENT: Parallel to the spinal cord and lateral margins of vertebral bodies

ANATOMIC COVERAGE: C7 to L1 and left to right lateral margins of vertebral bodies

TIP: "Anterior" saturation band (Sat A) in the field of view will help to compensate for breathing and aortic pulsation artifacts.
Superior and inferior sat bands (Sat S, Sat I) can help to compensate for CSF flow.

KEY: **CE**, cauda equina; **CM**, conus medularis; **HNP**, herniated nucleus pulposus; **InvD**, intervertebral disk; **PLL**, poster longitudinal ligament; **SC**, spinal cord; **SP**, spinous process.

Acquisition of Axial Image to Demonstrate Intervertebral Disk

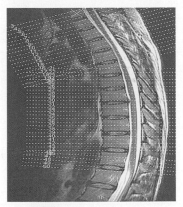

Figure 2-16 Sagittal image of the thoracic spine with axial locs

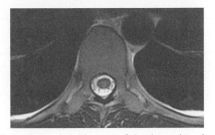

Figure 2-17 Axial image of the thoracic spine

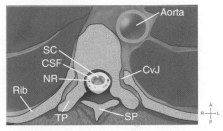

Figure 2-18 Axial anatomy of the thoracic spine

KEY: **CSF**, cerebral spinal fluid; **CvJ**, costovertebral joint; **NR**, nerve roots; **SC**, spinal cord; **SP**, spinous process; **TP**, transerve process

SLICE ACQUISITION: Superior to inferior, inferior C7 to superior L1

SLICE ALIGNMENT: For HNP: Parallel to intervertebral disk spaces in stacks of three to five slices

FOR OTHER PATHOLOGY: Multiple stacks parallel to vertebral bodies

ANATOMIC COVERAGE: From C7 through L1 vertebral body

Table 2-5   Thoracic Spine

Sequence 1.5	TR	TE	ETL or FA	Bandwidth	F Matrix	Ph Matrix	FOV	Slice Thick	Inter-Space	NEX	TI	Pulse Sequence Options
Sag. T2 FRFSE	3100	102	21	50	512	512	48/.60	3	1	2		Sat A, S-I, FC
Sag. T2 FSE	3500	102	25	41.67	448	224	32-36	3	1	4		Sat A, S-I, FC, NPW
Sag. T1 FSE	450	14	4	35.71	320	224	32-36	3	1	4		Sat A, TRF, NPW
Ax.T2 FRFSE	3300	110	27	41.67	256	224	20/.75	4	1	3		Sat A, S-I, FC, Zip 512
Ax.T1 FSE	550	Min	4	41.67	256	224	20/.75	5	0	3		Sat A, S-I
OPT Sag T2 FS	3500	85	27	41.67	320	224	32-36	3	1	2		Sat A, Fat, FC, NPW
Post GAD												
Ax.T1 FSE	550	Min	4	41.67	256	224	20/.75	5	0	3		Sat A, S-I
Sag. T1 FSE FS	525	14	4	31.25	320	224	32-36	3	1	4		Sat A, S-I, Fat, NPW, EDR

Table 2-5	Thoracic Spine—cont'd											
Sequence 3T	TR	TE	ETL or FA	Bandwidth	F Matrix	Ph Matrix	FOV	Slice Thick	Inter-Space	NEX	TI	Pulse Sequence Options
Sag. T2 FRFSE	3100	102	21	50	512	512	48/.60	3	1	2		Sat A, S-I, FC
Sag. T2 FSE	4000	110	21	50	416	224	32-36	3	.5	4		Sat A, S-I, FC, NPW
Sag.T1 Flair	3000	22	8	41.67	448	224	32-36	4	1	2	Auto	Sat S-I, A, seq, NPW
Ax.T2 FRFSE	5000	110	17	50	288	224	18/18	4	0	4		Sat A, FC, NPW

(Continued)

Table 2-5 Thoracic Spine—*cont'd*

Sequence 3T	TR	TE	ETL or FA	Bandwidth	F Matrix	Ph Matrix	FOV	Slice Thick	Inter-Space	NEX	TI	Pulse Sequence Options
Ax.T1 FSE	900	Min	4	62.50	256	224	18/18	5	0	2		Sat A, NPW, Zip 512
OPT Sag. T2 FS	3500	90	21	62.50	448	224	32-6	3	1	4		Sat A, S-I, Fat, FC, NPW
Post GAD												
Ax.T1 FSE	900	Min	4	62.50	256	224	18/18	5	0	2		Sat A, NPW, Zip 512
Sag.T1 Flair FS	3000	22	8	41.67	448	224	32-36	4	1	2	Auto	Sat S-I, A, Fat, Seq, NPW

Include the base of the brain through T-spine to count from C2.

T1 FSE ETL 4 or lower.

TRF (Tailor Radio-Frequency) should be used with all FSE sequences to increase # of slices per TR.

SPF (Swap phase and frequency) is used to reduce CSF artifacts. Use NPW when possibility of anatomy wrapping (No Phase Wrap).

Use IDEAL when available (see grab bag).

Table 2-6 Site Protocol: Thoracic Spine

Sequence 1.5	TR	TE	ETL or FA	Band-width	F Matrix	Ph Matrix	FOV	Slice Thick	Inter-space	NEX	TI	Pulse Sequence Options
Post GAD												

(Continued)

119

Table 2-6 Site Protocol: Thoracic Spine—*cont'd*

Sequence 3T	TR	TE	ETL or FA	Band-width	F Matrix	Ph Matrix	FOV	Slice Thick	Inter-space	NEX	TI	Pulse Sequence Options
Post GAD												

LUMBAR SPINE

Acquire three-plane pilot per site specifications.

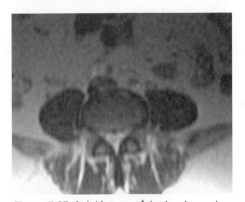

Figure 2-19 Axial image of the lumbar spine

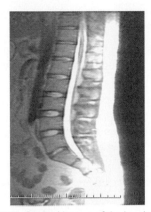

Figure 2-20 Sagittal image of the lumbar spine

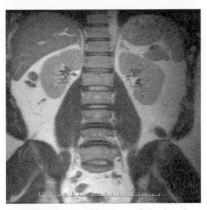

Figure 2-21 Coronal image of the lumbar spine

COIL: Multi-channel or HNS 4-5-6
POSITION: Supine, head first, cushion under knees
LANDMARK: Iliac crest
IMMOBILIZATION: Prevent body from touching sides of magnet by using sponges or sheets. Velcro bands may be used across the torso.

TIP: Contrast is indicated in postoperative lumbar spine to differentiate recurrent HNP vs. scar tissue.

Acquisition of Sagittal Images of the Lumbar Spine

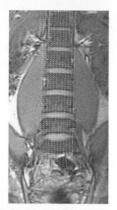

Figure 2-22 Coronal image of the lumbar spine with sagittal locations

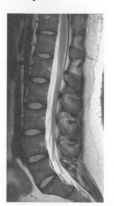

Figure 2-23 Sagittal image of lumbar spine with anterior saturation band

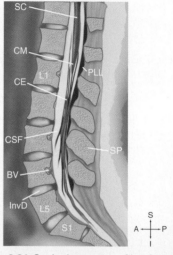

Figure 2-24 Sagittal anatomy of lumbar spine

SLICE ACQUISITION: Left to right
SLICE ALIGNMENT: Parallel to left and right lateral margins of vertebral bodies
ANATOMIC COVERAGE: Left transverse process to right transverse process, T12 to sacrum

TIPS: Anterior saturation band (Sat A) in the field of view will help to compensate for breathing and peristalsis artifacts.
Superior and inferior sat bands (Sat S, Sat I) can help to compensate for CSF flow.

KEY: **BV,** basilar vein; **CE,** cauda equina; **CM,** conus medularis; **CSF,** cerebral spinal fluid; **InvD,** intervertebral disk; **PLL,** poster longitudinal ligament; **SC,** spinal cord; **SP,** spinous process.

Acquisition of Axial Images

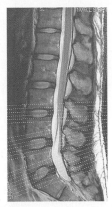

Figure 2-25 Sagittal image of the lumbar spine with axial locs and anterior saturation band

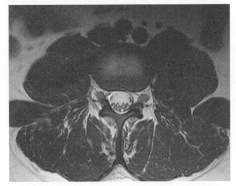

Figure 2-26 Axial image of the lumbar spine

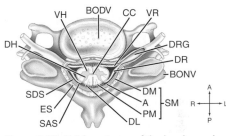

Figure 2-27 Axial anatomy of the lumbar spine

KEY: **A**, arachnoid; **BODV**, body of vertebra; **BONV**, bone of vertebra; **CC**, central canal; **DH**, dorsal horn; **DL**, denticulate ligaments; **DM**, dura mater (spinal dural sheath); **DR**, dorsal root; **DRG**, dorsal root ganglion; **ES**, epidural space (contains fat); **SAS**, subarachnoid space; **SDS**, subdural space; **SM**, spinal meninges; **VH**, ventral horn; **VR**, ventral root.

SLICE ACQUISITION: Superior to inferior

SLICE ALIGNMENT: Parallel to intervertebral disk spaces

ANATOMIC COVERAGE: For HNP, align to disk spaces from L1 to S1. For other pathology, contiguous slices angled through vertebral bodies should be performed.

| Table 2-7 | | | | | | | | | | | | Routine Lumbar Spine |

Sequence 1.5	TR	TE	ETL or FA	Band-width	F Matrix	Ph Matrix	FOV	Slice Thick	Inter-Space	NEX	TI	Pulse Sequence Options
Sag. T2 FRFSE	3500	110	27	50	448	224	28-30	4	1	4		Sat A, S-I, FC, NPW
Sag. T1 FSE	600	Min	2	35.71	320	224	28-30	4	1	2		Sat A, NPW
Ax.T2 FRFSE	3400	102	15	41.67	256	224	20/20	4	1	3		Sat A, S-I, FC, Zip 512
Ax.T1 FSE	550	Min	4	41.67	256	224	20/.75	4	1	2		Sat A, S-I, Zip 512
OPT Sag T2 FS	3500	85	27	41.67	320	224	28-30	3	1	2		Sat A, Fat, FC, NPW
Post GAD												
Ax.T1 FSE	600	Min	4	41.67	256	224	20/20	4	1	2		Sat A, S-I, Zip 512
Sag. T1 FS	600	Min	4	31.25	320	224	28-30	4	1	2		Sat A, S-I, Fat, NPW

Table 2-7 Thoracic Spine—*cont'd*

Sequence 3T	TR	TE	ETL or FA	Band-width	F Matrix	Ph Matrix	FOV	Slice Thick	Inter-Space	NEX	TI	Pulse Sequence Options
Sag. T2 FRFSE	4300	102	23	50	448	224	26-30	3	1	4		FRFSE, Sat A, S-I, FC, TRF, NPW
Sag. T1 Flair	3000	22	8	41.67	448	224	26-30	4	1	2	Auto	Sat S-I, A, Seq, NPW
Ax. T2 FRFSE	5200	110	23	50	320	224	18/18	4	.5	4		Sat A, FC, NPW
Ax. T1 FSE	900	Min	4	41.67	320	224	18/18	4	.5	2		Sat A, S-I, Zip 512
OPT Sag. T2 FS	3500	102	25	50	448	224	26-30	4	1	2		Sat Fat, A, S-I, FC, NPW
Post GAD												
Ax. T1	900	Min	4	41.67	320	224	18/18	4	.5	2		Sat A, S-I, Zip 512
Sag. T1 Flair FS	3000	22	8	41.67	448	224	26-30	4	1	2	Auto	Fast, Sat S-I, A, Fat, seq, NPW

T1 FSE ETL 4 or lower.
TRF (Tailor Radio-Frequency) should be used with all FSE sequences to increase # of slices per TR.
Use NPW when possibility of anatomy wrapping (No Phase Wrap).
Use IDEAL when available (see grab bag).

Table 2-8 Site Protocol: Lumbar Spine

Sequence 1.5	TR	TE	ETL or FA	Band-width	F Matrix	Ph Matrix	FOV	Slice Thick	Inter-space	NEX	TI	Pulse Sequence Options
Post GAD												

Sequence 3T	TR	TE	ETL or FA	Band-width	F Matrix	Ph Matrix	FOV	Slice Thick	Inter-space	NEX	TI	Pulse Sequence Options
Post GAD												

Table 2-8 Site Protocol: Lumbar Spine—*cont'd*

SACROILIAC JOINTS—SACRUM AND COCCYX

Acquire three-plane pilot per site specifications.

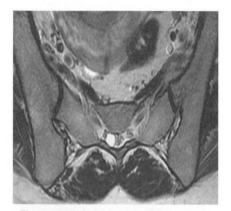
Figure 2-28 Axial image of the sacrum

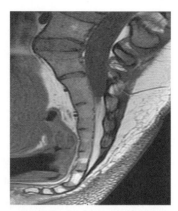
Figure 2-29 Sagittal image of the sacrum

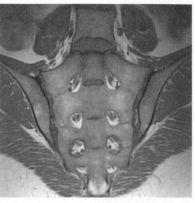
Figure 2-30 Coronal image of the sacrum

COIL: Multi-channel or HNS 4-5-6

POSITION: Supine, head first, cushion under knees

LANDMARK: ASIS

IMMOBILIZATION: Prevent the body from touching the sides of the magnet by using sponges or sheets. Velcro bands may be used across the torso.

Acquisition of Coronal Image of Sacroiliac Joints: Sacrum and Coccyx

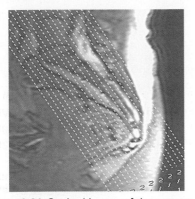

Figure 2-31 Sagittal image of the sacrum with coronal locations

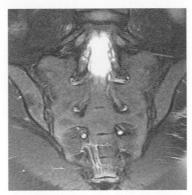

Figure 2-32 Coronal image of the sacrum

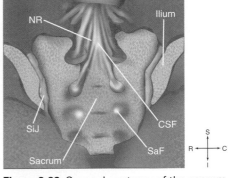

Figure 2-33 Coronal anatomy of the sacrum

KEY: CSF, cerebral spinal fluid; **NR**, nerve roots; **SaF**, sacral foramen; **SiJ**, sacroiliac joint.

SLICE ACQUISITION: Anterior to posterior

SLICE ALIGNMENT: Parallel to sacrum

ANATOMIC COVERAGE: Body of the sacrum to include the left and right sacroiliac joints as referenced on coronal location.

TIP: Sat A in the field of view can help to compensate for peristalsis and vascular motion. When performing an examination for the coccyx, copy and paste coronal parameters and perform in the sagittal plane.

Acquisition of Axial Image of Sacroiliac Joints: Sacrum and Coccyx

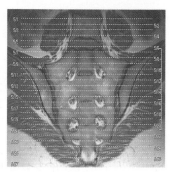

Figure 2-34 Coronal image of the sacrum with axial locations

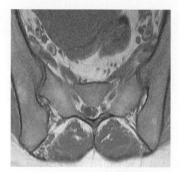

Figure 2-35 Axial image of the sacrum

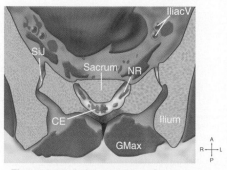

Figure 2-36 Axial anatomy of the sacrum

KEY: **CE**, cauda equina; **GMax**, gluteus maximus; **SiJ**, sacroiliac joint; **NR**, nerve roots.

SLICE ACQUISITION: Superior to inferior

SLICE ALIGNMENT: Parallel to sacral body

ANATOMIC COVERAGE: From inferior body of L5 through the sacrum; include the coccyx when indicated.

Table 2-9 Sacroiliac Joints and Sacrum and Coccyx

Sequence 1.5	TR	TE	ETL or FA	Band-width	F Matrix	Ph Matrix	FOV	Slice Thick	Inter-Space	NEX	TI	Pulse Sequence Options
Cor T2 FRFSE FS	3500	110	19	41.67	448	224	26/26	4	1	4		Sat A, FAT FC, NPW
Cor T1 FSE	500	Min	4	31.25	256	224	26/26	4	1	2		Sat A, NPW, EDR, ZIP 512
Ax.T2 FRFSE	3400	102	11	41.67	256	224	20/20	4	1.5	4		Sat A, S-I, FC, NPW, Zip 512
Ax.T1 FSE	600	Min	4	31.25	320	224	20/20	4	1.5	2		Sat A, S-I, NPW, Zip 512
Post GAD												
Ax.T1 FSE FS	600	Min	4	31.25	320	224	20/20	4	1.5	2		Sat A, S-I, NPW, Zip 512
Cor T1 FSE FS	500	Min	4	31.25	256	224	26/26	4	1	2		Sat A, NPW, EDR, ZIP 512

(Continued)

Table 2-9	Sacroiliac Joints and Sacrum and Coccyx—*cont'd*											
Sequence 3T	**TR**	**TE**	**ETL or FA**	**Band-width**	**F Matrix**	**Ph Matrix**	**FOV**	**Slice Thick**	**Inter-Space**	**NEX**	**TI**	**Pulse Sequence Options**
Cor T2 FRFSE FS	4300	102	23	41.67	512	288	26/26	4	1	4		Sat A, Fat, FC, NPW
Cor.T1 FSE	900	Min	4	41.67	320	224	26/26	4	1	2		Sat A, S-I, Zip 512
Ax.T2 FRFSE	4800	110	23	41.67	320	224	18/18	4	1.5	4		Sat A, FC, NPW
Ax.T1 FSE	900	Min	4	41.67	320	224	18/18	4	1.5	2		Sat A, S-I, NPW, Zip 512
Post GAD												
Ax.T1 FSE FS	900	Min	4	41.67	320	224	18/18	4	1.5	2		Sat A, Fat, FC, Zip 512
Cor.T1 FSE FS	900	Min	4	41.67	320	224	26/26	4	1	2		Sat A, Fat, FC, Zip 512

T1 FSE ETL 4 of lower.
TRF (Tailor Radio-Frequency) should be used with all FSE sequences to increase # of slices per TR.
Use NPW when possibility of anatomy wrapping (No Phase Wrap).
Use IDEAL when available (see grab bag).
When performing exam for coccyx, copy and paste coronal parameters and perform in the sagittal plane.

Table 2-10 Site Protocol: Sacroiliac Joints and Sacrum and Coccyx

Sequence 1.5	TR	TE	ETL or FA	Band-width	F Matrix	Ph Matrix	FOV	Slice Thick	Inter-space	NEX	TI	Pulse Sequence Options
Post GAD												

Sequence 3T	TR	TE	ETL or FA	Band-width	F Matrix	Ph Matrix	FOV	Slice Thick	Inter-space	NEX	TI	Pulse Sequence Options
Post GAD												

MRI OF THE BONY PELVIS

Acquire three-plane pilot per site specifications.

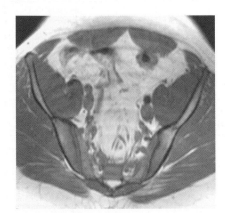

Figure 2-37 Axial image of the pelvis

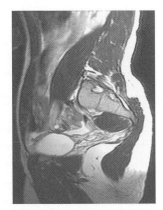

Figure 2-38 Sagittal image of the pelvis

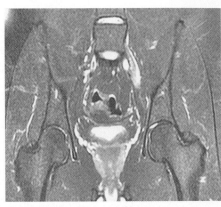

Figure 2-39 Coronal image of the pelvis

COIL: Multi-channel torso coil
POSITION: Supine feet first, with legs flat and extended. Use cushions to avoid rotation of the pelvis. Place a cushion between the ankles, with tape securing feet in 15-degree internal rotation.
LANDMARK: ASIS
IMMOBILIZATION: Place hands on the chest, which may be secured with Velcro straps.
   Prevent the body from touching the sides of the magnet by using sponges or sheets.

Acquisition of Coronal Image

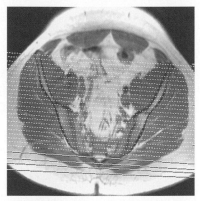

Figure 2-40 Axial image of the pelvis with coronal locations

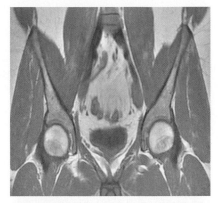

Figure 2-41 Coronal image of the pelvis

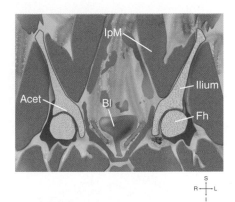

Figure 2-42 Coronal anatomy of the pelvis

KEY: **Acet**, acetebellum; **Bl**, bladder; **Fh**, femoral head; **IpM**, iliopsoas muscle.

SLICE ACQUISITION: Anterior to posterior
SLICE ALIGNMENT: Perpendicular to bilateral ASIS
ANATOMIC COVERAGE: From anterior ASIS to posterior sacrum

TIP: Anterior saturation band (saturation A) in the field of view will help to compensate for respiration, peristalsis, and vascular motion.

Acquisition of Axial Image

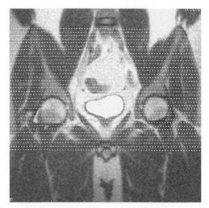

Figure 2-43 Coronal image of the pelvis with axial locations

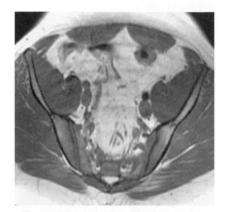

Figure 2-44 Axial image of the pelvis

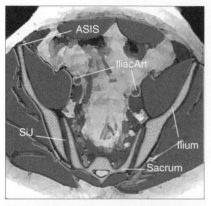

Figure 2-45 Axial anatomy of the pelvis

SLICE ACQUISITION: Superior to inferior
SLICE ALIGNMENT: Parallel to bilateral iliac crest
ANATOMIC COVERAGE: Iliac crest to ischial ramus to include the ala bilaterally

KEY: **FN**, fermoral nerve; **I**, ilium; **IM**, iliacus muscle; **IS**, ischial spine; **OIM**, obturator internus muscle; **P**, pubis; **PM**, piriformis muscle; **PMM**, psoas major muscle; **SIJ**, sacroiliac joints; **S**, sacrum.

Table 2-11 Routine Bony Pelvis

Sequence 1.5	TR	TE	ETL or FA	Band-width	F Matrix	Ph Matrix	FOV	Slice Thick	Inter-Space	NEX	TI	Pulse Sequence Options
Cor T2 FRFSE FS	3500	110	19	41.67	448	224	36-44	4	1	4		Sat S-I, Fat FC
Cor T1 FSE	500	Min	4	31.25	256	224	36-44	4	1	2		Sat S-I, EDR, ZIP 512
Ax.T2 FRFSE FS	3400	102	11	41.67	256	224	36-44	4	1.5	4		Sat A, Fat, FC
Ax.T1 FSE	600	Min	4	31.25	320	224	36-44	4	1.5	2		Sat A, S-I, Zip 512
Post GAD												
Ax.T1 FSE FS	600	Min	4	31.25	320	224	36-44	4	1.5	2		Sat A, S-I, Zip 512
Cor T1 FSE FS	500	Min	4	31.25	256	224	36-44	4	1	2		Sat A, Fat, ZIP 512

(Continued)

Table 2-11 Routine Bony Pelvis—*cont'd*

Sequence 3T	TR	TE	ETL or FA	Band-width	F Matrix	Ph Matrix	FOV	Slice Thick	Inter-Space	NEX	TI	Pulse Sequence Options
Cor T2 FRFSE FS	4300	102	23	41.67	448	288	36-44	4	1	4		Sat S-I Fat, FC
Cor.T1 FSE	900	Min	4	41.67	320	224	36-44	4	1	2		Sat S-I, Zip 512
Ax.T2 FRFSE FS	4800	110	23	41.67	320	224	36-44	4	1.5	4		Sat A, Fat, FC
Ax.T1 FSE	900	Min	4	41.67	320	224	36-44	4	1.5	2		Sat A, S-I, Zip 512
Post GAD												
Ax.T1 FSE FS	900	Min	4	41.67	320	224	36-44	4	.5	2		Sat A, Fat, FC, Zip 512
Cor FSE T1 FS	900	Min	4	41.67	320	224	36-44	4	1	2		Sat A, Fat, FC, Zip 512

T1 FSE ETL 4 of lower.
TRF (Tailor Radio-Frequency) should be used with all FSE sequences to increase # of slices per TR.
Use NPW when possibility of anatomy wrapping (No Phase Wrap).
Use IDEAL when available (see grab bag).

Table 2-12 Site Protocol: Bony Pelvis

Sequence 1.5	TR	TE	ETL or FA	Band-width	F Matrix	Ph Matrix	FOV	Slice Thick	Inter-space	NEX	TI	Pulse Sequence Options
Post GAD												

Sequence 3T	TR	TE	ETL or FA	Band-width	F Matrix	Ph Matrix	FOV	Slice Thick	Inter-space	NEX	TI	Pulse Sequence Options
Post GAD												

MR Myelography of the Spine

Myelography can be acquired in addition to MRI of the spine in the cervical, thoracic or lumbar regions.

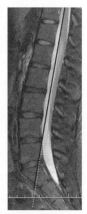

Figure 2-46 Sagittal of the lumbar spine with loc for lumbar myelogram

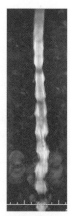

Figure 2-47 Myelogram image of the lumbar spine

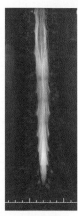

Figure 2-48 Myelogram image of thoracic spine

MR Myelography is a high contrast imaging technique which visualizes CSF surrounding the spinal cord and adjacent structures. It uses a High TR-TE technique which resembles a traditional Myelogram. This technique suppresses all tissue while visualizing CSF as bright because of its long relaxation time. See Grab Bag (Table 2-13) for suggested technique.

COIL: CTL or HNS
POSITITON: Supine, head first, cushion under knees
LANDMARK: Appropriate to region of the spine

Table 2-13 Grab Bag

Sequence 1.5	TR	TE	ETL or FA	Band-width	F Matrix	Ph Matrix	FOV	Slice Thick	Inter-space	NEX	TI	Pulse Sequence Options
IDEAL T1	667	14	3-4	31.25	256	192		3	1	2		IDEAL, Fast, ZIP 512, TRF
IDEAL T2	3500	85	29	62.5	256	224		3	1	2		IDEAL, Fast, ZIP 512, TRF, NPW
MYLEO	6000-9000	950		62.5	384	192	24-36	20-50	0	.53		SSFSE, FC, Sat F
MYLEO HR	7000-9000	950	48	31.25	512	512	24-36/.80	20-50	0	1		FRFSE, FC, Sat F, TRF

(Continued)

Table 2-13	Grab Bag—*cont'd*											
Sequence 3T	TR	TE	ETL or FA	Band-width	F Matrix	Ph Matrix	FOV	Slice Thick	Inter-space	NEX	TI	Pulse Sequence Options
IDEAL T1	850	Min full	3-4	62.5	320	192		3	1	2		IDEAL, Fast, ZIP 512, TRF
IDEAL T2	4250	110	20	62.5	256	224		3	1	2		IDEAL, Fast, ZIP 512, TRF, NPW
MYLEO	7000-9000	950		83.33	320	24-36	24-36	20-50	0	.53		SSFSE, FC, Sat F
MYLEO HR	7000-9000	950	48	50	512	512	24-36/.80	20-50	0	1		FRFSE, FC, Sat F, TRF

TRF (Tailor Radio-Frequency) should be used with all FSE sequences to increase # of slices per TR.
Use NPW when possbility of anatomy wrapping (No Phase Wrap).
FOV for MYLEO is dependent on the spine location of interest.

Table 2-14 Site Protocol: Grab Bag

Sequence 1.5	TR	TE	ETL/FA	Band-width	F Matix	Ph Matrix	FOV	Slice Thick	Inter-space	NEX	TI	Pulse Sequence Options
Post GAD												

(Continued)

Table 2-14 Site Protocol: Grab Bag—*cont'd*

Sequence 3T	TR	TE	ETL/FA	Band-width	F Matix	Ph Matrix	FOV	Slice Thick	Inter-space	NEX	TI	Pulse Sequence Options
Post GAD												

MRI of the Upper Extremities

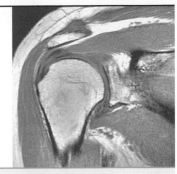

CHAPTER OUTLINE

MRI OF THE UPPER EXTREMITIES—CONSIDERATIONS

Scan Considerations

- Extremities should be scanned in the anatomical position when possible. Consider the patient's tolerance for pain: a neutral position may be necessary.
- When scanning long bones, it may be difficult to fit the anatomy into a single coil. Repositioning the patient may be required.
- Place a vitamin E capsule or MRI-compatible marker at the area of pain or interest.
- Refer to all safety-related parameters.
- As the SAR (specific absorption rate) increases, the patient's body temperature will also increase. SAR elevation can be compensated for by increasing the TR slightly. If this is not done correctly at 3T, the SAR will increase and the scanner will stop as a patient safety precaution. All 3T systems have SAR monitors, which should be referenced while scanning. This is not an issue at 1.5T.
- Contrast is often used for osteomyelitis, tumor, or infection.
- MR arthrogram is performed to best demonstrate labral pathology. Arthrography of the shoulder is performed to demonstrate labrum pathology of the shoulder. In the elbow, it is performed to for intra-articular body evaluation or medial or lateral collateral ligament pathology. A mixture of gadolinium and iodinated contrast is injected into the bursa in a fluoroscopy suite before the MRI is performed.
- Orthopedic hardware can cause distortion and metallic artefacts in the image. To help compensate, the bandwidth should be increased, the ETL can be increased, and the NEX (number of excitations) can be increased. These options will help but not eliminate these artefact.

Coils

- Multi-channel body-specific coils are used when available. Any coil that covers the anatomy may be used, i.e., the knee coil may be used to scan the elbow.
- All multi-channel coils produce excessive signal adjacent to the coil. This can be compensated for by using vendor-specific options to provide uniform signal intensity.

Pulse Sequences

- T1 is used to best identify anatomic structures, whereas T2 fat saturation (FS) and or STIR (short T1 inversion recovery) provides detailed evidence of pathology.
- On T1 sequences, bone should appear bright or hyperintense because fat in the bone has a short relaxation time. On T1 sequences, fluid will appear dark or hypointense because water has a long T1 relaxation time.
- On T2 sequences, fluid produces bright or hyperintense signal as a result of long T2 relaxation. Musculoskeletal (MSK) T2 imaging uses fat saturation or STIR to eliminate the fat and enhance abnormal fluid of pathology in bone.
- T1 FS are used post routine arthrogram to best visualize the contrast in the joint. T2 FS may also be added.
- T1 and/or T2 CUBE can be used to obtain high-resolution sub-millimeter images of the wrist.

Options

- Fat saturation (FS) options and terminology are vendor specific. For GE systems, use "fat classic" for fat saturation with enhanced anatomical detail.
- IDEAL (GE) is a fat/water separation technique (previously called 3-point Dixon technique). This technique eliminates fat and water and provides an in and out of phase image, all in one acquisition. IDEAL can be used with T1, T2, and SPGR when imaging extremities.
- Superior and inferior saturation bands help to compensate for vascular pulsation, whereas left or right saturation bands can help compensate for breathing or cardiac motion. Saturation bands can be used on all pulse sequences.
- Flow compensation (FC) or gradient nulling should be used on T2 images to help compensate for vascular motion.

MRI OF THE SHOULDER

Acquire a three-plane pilot per site specifications.

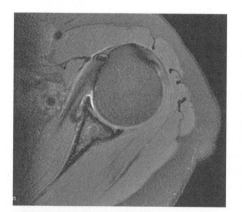

Figure 3-1 Axial image of the shoulder

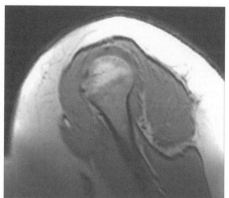

Figure 3-2 Sagittal image of the shoulder

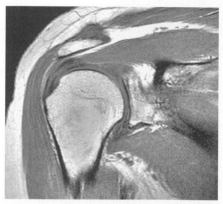

Figure 3-3 Coronal image of the shoulder

COIL: Multi-channel shoulder coil is preferred.

POSITION: Supine, head first, cushion under the patient's knees. Arm on affected side extended and hand placed at patient's side, palm up when possible

LANDMARK: Coracoid process

IMMOBILIZATION: Cushion under humerus to support arm. Velcro strap across torso to secure limb during scan if needed.

TIP: Position shoulder as close to isocenter as possible.

For arthrogram, follow same protocol as for routine shoulder, and refer to Table 3-3 for scan parameters.

Acquisition of Axial Images

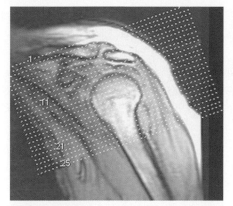

Figure 3-4 Coronal image of the shoulder with axial locations

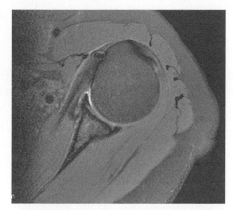

Figure 3-5 Axial image of the shoulder

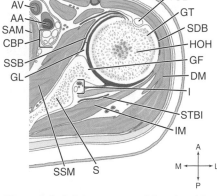

Figure 3-6 Axial anatomy of the shoulder

SLICE ACQUISITION: Superior to inferior

SLICE ALIGNMENT: Perpendicular to shaft and head of humerus

ANATOMIC COVERAGE: From above acromioclavicular joint through surgical neck of humerus

TIP: Left or right saturation band in the field to eliminate heart and breathing motion. Include the entire acromioclavicular joint to demonstrate possible pathologic condition.

KEY: **AA**, axillary artery; **AV**, axillary vein; **CBP**, cords of brachial plexus; **DM**, deltoid muscle; **GF**, glenoid fossa; **GL**, glenoid labrum; **GT**, greater tuberosity; **HOH**, head of humerus; **I**, infraspinatus; **IM**, infraspinatus muscle; **S**, scapula; **SDB**, subdeltoid (subacromial) bursa; **SSB**, subscapularis bursa; **SSM**, subscapularis muscle; **STBI**, subtendinous bursa of infraspinatus; **TOB**, tendon of biceps.

Acquisition of Coronal Images

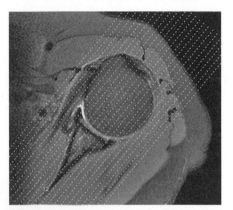

Figure 3-7 Axial image of the shoulder with coronal locations

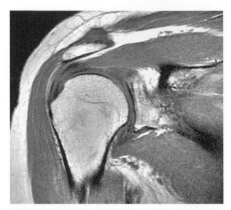

Figure 3-8 Coronal image of the shoulder

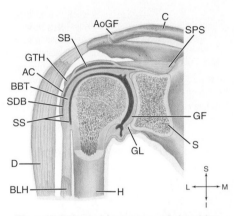

Figure 3-9 Coronal anatomy of shoulder

SLICE ACQUISITION: Anterior to posterior
SLICE ALIGNMENT: Perpendicular to the glenoid fossa, parallel to supraspinatus muscle
ANATOMICAL COVERAGE: Subscapularis muscle through the supraspinatus tendon

TIP: Left or right saturation band in the FOV to eliminate heart and breathing motion.

KEY: **AC**, articular capsule; **AoGF**, acromion on glenoid fossa; **BBT**, biceps brachii tendon; **BLH**, biceps, long head; **C**, clavicle; **D**, deltoid; **GF**, glenoid fossa; **GL**, glenoid labrum; **GTH**, greater tubercle of humerus; **H**, humerus; **S**, scapula; **SB**, subacromial bursa; **SDB**, subdeltoid bursa; **SS**, synovial sheath; **SPS**, supraspinatus.

Acquisition of Sagittal Images

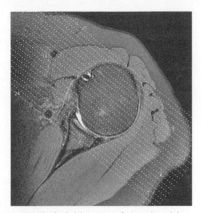

Figure 3-10 Axial image of the shoulder with sagittal locations

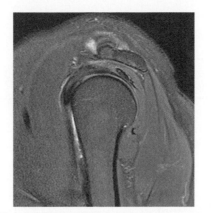

Figure 3-11 Sagittal image of the shoulder

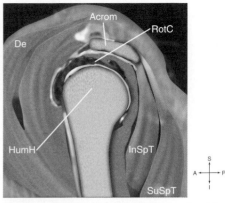

Figure 3-12 Sagittal anatomy of the shoulder

SLICE ACQUISITION: Lateral to medial
SLICE ALIGNMENT: Parallel to the glenoid fossa
ANATOMIC COVERAGE: Entire deltoid muscle through glenoid fossa

KEY: **Acrom**, acromion; **De**, deltoid; **HumH**, hemoral head; **InSpT**, infraspinatus tendon; **RotC**, rotator cuff; **SuSpT**, supraspinatus tendon.

151

Table 3-1 Routine Shoulder

Sequence 1.5	TR	TE	ETL or FA	Band-width	F Matrix	Ph Matrix	FOV	Slice Thick	Inter-space	NEX	TI	Pulse Sequence Options
AX PD FRFSE FS	2400	30	7	31.25	256	224	15/15	3	.5	4		Sat L or R, F, FC, NPW
Cor PD FS FSE	2600	30	7	31.25	256	224	15/15	3	.3	4		Sat L or R, F, FC, NPW
Cor T2 FRFSE FS	3500	68	11	31.25	256	224	15/15	3	.3	4		Sat L or R, F, FC, NPW
Cor T1 FSE	650	Min	3	31.25	256	224	15/15	3	.3	4		Sat L or R, NPW
Sag T2 FSE	3200	68	7	31.25	256	224	15/15	3	.3	4		Sat L or R, FC, NPW, Zip 512
OPT Sag T2 FS	3500	68	27	31.25	256	224	15/15	3	.3	4		Sat L or R, F, FC, NPW, Zip 512

Table 3-1 Routine Shoulder—*cont'd*

Sequence 3T	TR	TE	ETL or FA	Band-width	F Matrix	Ph Matrix	FOV	Slice Thick	Inter-space	NEX	TI	Pulse Sequence Options
Ax PD FRFSE FS	2500	32	7	50	288	224	14/14	3	.5	3		Sat L or R, F, FC, NPW
Cor PD FSE FS	3300	Min	7	50	320	224	14/14	3	0	2		Sat L or R, F, FC, TRF
Cor T2 FRFSE FS	5800	80	18	50	320	224	14/14	3	0	2		Sat L or R, Fat, FC, NPW
Cor T1 FSE	1100	Min	4	50	320	224	14/14	3	0	3		Sat L or R, NPW
Sag T2 FRFSE	3000	68	17	50	288	224	14/14	3	0	3		Sat L or R, F, FC, NPW, Zip 512
OPT Sag T2 FS	3000	68	17	50	288	224	14/14	3	0	3		Sat L or R, Fat, FC, NPW, Zip 512
Ax PD FRFSE FS	2400	30	7	31.25	256	224	15/15	3	.5	4		Sat L or R, F, FC, NPW
Cor PD FS FSE	2600	30	7	31.25	256	224	15/15	3	.3	4		Sat L or R, F, FC, NPW

T1 FSE ETL 4 of lower.
TRF (Tailor Radio-Frequency) should be used with all FSE sequences to increase # of slices per TR.
Use NPW when possibility of anatomy wrapping (No Phase Wrap).
IDEAL can be used available (see grab bag in spine section).

Table 3-2   Site Protocol: Routine Shoulder

Sequence 1.5	TR	TE	ETL or FA	Band-width	F Matrix	Ph Matrix	FOV	Slice Thick	Inter-space	NEX	TI	Pulse Sequence Options

Sequence 3T	TR	TE	ETL or FA	Band width	F Matrix	Ph Matrix	FOV	Slice Thick	Inter-space	NEX	TI	Pulse Sequence Options

| Table 3-3 | Routine Arthrogram of Shoulder |

Sequence 1.5	TR	TE	ETL/ FA	Band-width	F Matrix	Ph Matrix	FOV	Slice Thick	Inter-space	NEX	TI	Pulse Sequence Options
Ax T1 FSE FS	650	Min	3	31.25	256	224	14/14	3	.3	4		Sat F, L or R, NPW
Cor T1 FSE FS	650	Min	3	31.25	256	224	14/14	3	.3	4		Sat F, L or R, NPW
Sag T1 FSE FS	650	Min	3	31.25	256	224	14/14	3	.3	4		Sat F, L or R, NPW
Cor T2 FRFSE FS	3500	68	11	31.25	256	224	14/14	3	.3	4		Sat L or R, Fat, FC, NPW
Ax 3-D FGRE	Mach	Min	20	31.25	256	192	14/14	3	40loc/ slab	2	250	IRP, Zip 512, Zip 2

(Continued)

Table 3-3 Routine Arthrogram of Shoulder—*cont'd*

Sequence 3T	TR	TE	ETL/ FA	Band-width	F Matrix	Ph Matrix	FOV	Slice Thick	Inter-space	NEX	TI	Pulse Sequence Options
Ax T1 FSE FS	1100	Min	4	50	320	224	14/14	3	0	3		Sat F, L or R, NPW
Cor T1 FSE FS	1100	Min	4	50	320	224	14/14	3	0	3		Sat F, L or R, NPW
Sag T1 FSE FS	1100	Min	4	50	320	224	14/14	3	0	3		Sat F, L or R, NPW
Cor T2 FRFSE FS	5800	80	18	50	320	224	14/14	3	0	2		Sat L or R, Fat, FC, NPW
Ax 3-D FGRE	Mach	Min	20	31.25	256	192	14/14	3	40 loc/ slab	1	450	IRP, Zip 512, Zip 2

FSE ETL 4 of lower.

TRF (Tailor Radio-Frequency) should be used with all FSE sequences to increase # of slices per TR.

Use NPW when possbility of anatomy wrapping (No Phase Wrap).

IDEAL can be used available (see grab bag in spine).

Table 3-4 Site Protocol: Routine Arthrogram of Shoulder

Sequence 1.5	TR	TE	ETL/ FA	Band-width	F Matrix	Ph Matrix	FOV	Slice Thick	Inter-space	NEX	TI	Pulse Sequence Options

(Continued)

Table 3-4 Site Protocol: Routine Arthrogram of Shoulder—*cont'd*

Sequence 3T	TR	TE	ETL/ FA	Band-width	F Matrix	Ph Matrix	FOV	Slice Thick	Inter-space	NEX	TI	Pulse Sequence Options

MRI OF THE HUMERUS

Acquire three-plane pilot per site specifications.

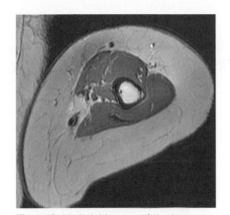

Figure 3-13 Axial image of the humerus

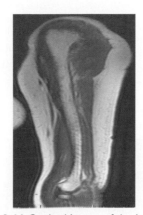

Figure 3-14 Sagittal image of the humerus

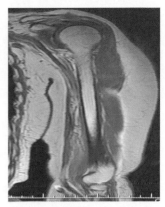

Figure 3-15 Coronal image of the humerus

COIL: Multi-channel torso or cardiac coil, depending on patient size

POSITION: Supine, head first, cushion under the patient's knees

Position the patient to place the arm as close to the isocenter as possible; arm should be resting at patient's side, palm up when possible.

LANDMARK: Midshaft of the humerus

IMMOBILIZATION: Cushion under the humerus so shaft is in the same plane as the shoulder. Secure arm with Velcro strap.

TIP: Occasionally, two studies must be performed to ensure adequate resolution to demonstrate both the shoulder and elbow joint.

Acquisition of Axial Images of the Humerus

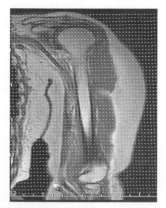

Figure 3-16 Coronal image of the humerus with axial locations

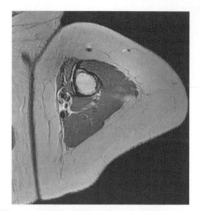

Figure 3-17 Axial image of the humerus

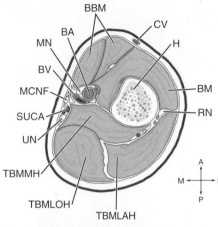

Figure 3-18 Axial anatomy of the humerus

SLICE ACQUISITION: Superior to inferior
SLICE ALIGNMENT: Perpendicular to the shaft of the humerus
ANATOMIC COVERAGE: Humeral head through elbow joint

KEY: **BA**, brachial artery; **BBM**, biceps brachii muscle; **BM**, brachialis muscle; **BV**, basiliar vein; **CV**, cephalic vein; **H**, humerus; **MCNF**, medial cutaneous nerve of forearm; **MN**, median nerve; **RN**, radial nerve; **SUCA**, superior ulnar collateral artery; **TBMLAH**, triceps brachii muscle, lateral head; **TBMLOH**, triceps brachii muscle, long head; **TBMMH**, triceps brachii muscle, medial head; **UN**, ulnar nerve.

Acquisition of Coronal Images of the Humerus

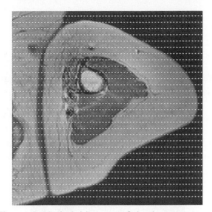

Figure 3-19 Axial image of the humerus with coronal locations

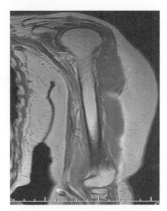

Figure 3-20 Coronal image of the humerus

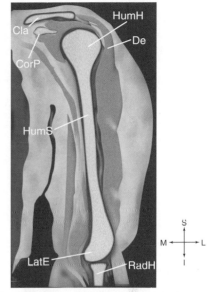

Figure 3-21 Coronal anatomy of the humerus

SLICE ACQUISITION: Anterior to posterior

SLICE ALIGNMENT: Parallel to shaft of the humerus

ANATOMIC COVERAGE: Entire humerus, including shoulder and elbow joint

KEY: **Cla**, clavicle; **Corp**, corocoid process; **De**, deltoid muscle; **HumH**, humeral head; **HumS**, humeral shaft; **LatE**, lateral epicondyle; **RadH**, radial head.

Acquisition of Sagittal Images of the Humerus

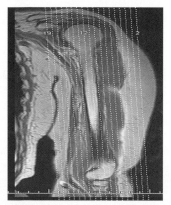

Figure 3-22 Coronal image of the humerus with sagittal locations

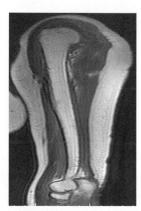

Figure 3-23 Sagittal image of the humerus

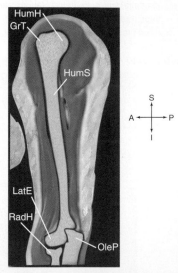

Figure 3-24 Sagittal anatomy of the humerus

SLICE ACQUISITION: Lateral to medial
SLICE ALIGNMENT: Parallel to shaft of humerus
ANATOMIC COVERAGE: Entire humerus including the shoulder and elbow joint

KEY: **GrT,** greater tubercule; **HumH,** humeral head; **HumS,** humeral shaft; **LatE,** lateral epicondyle; **OleP,** olecranon process; **RadH,** radial head.

Table 3-5 Routine Humerus

Sequence 1.5	TR	TE	ETL or FA	Band-width	F Matrix	Ph Matrix	FOV	Slice Thick	Inter-space	NEX	TI	Pulse Sequence Options
Cor T1 FSE	500	Min	4	31.25	320	224	30/.75	3	1	3		Sat S-I, NPW
Cor IR FSE	4000	42	7	31.25	256	192	30/.75	3	1	2	150	Sat S-I, FC, seq, NPW
Ax PD FSE	3000	30	10	31.25	256	224	12-14	5	.5-1	3		Sat S-I, FC, NPW
Ax T2 FSE FS	3500	65	11	41.67	256	192	12-14	5	.5-1	3		Sat S-I, F, FC, TRF, NPW
Sag T2 FRFSE FS	3500	60	9	41.67	256	192	30/.75	3	1	2		Sat S-I, F, FC
OPT Sag FSE IR	4000	42		31.25	256	192	30/.75	3	1	2	150	Sat S-I, FC, seq

(Continued)

Table 3-5												Routine Humerus—*cont'd*

Sequence 3T	TR	TE	ETL or FA	Band-width	F Matrix	Ph Matrix	FOV	Slice Thick	Inter-space	NEX	TI	Pulse Sequence Options
Cor T1 FSE	1200	20	3	41.67	384	224	30/.75	3	0	2		Sat S-I, NPW
Cor IR FSE	4000	42	25	41.67	256	192	30/.75	3	0	2	190	Sat S-I, FC, seq, NPW
Ax PD FSE	3000	30	10	31.25	256	224	12-14	5	.5-1	3		Sat S-I, FC, NPW
Ax T2 FS	3500	65	15	50	320	224	15/15	5	.5-1	2		Sat S-I, FC, NPW
Sag T2 FRFSE FS	4000	60	15	41.67	320	224	30/.75	3	0	2		Sat S-I, F, FC
OPT Sag FSE IR	4000	42		41.67	256	224	30/.75	3	0	2	190	Sat S-I, FC, seq

FSE ETL 4 of lower.

TRF (Tailor Radio-Frequency) should be used with all FSE sequences to increase # of slices per TR.

Use NPW when possibility of anatomy wrapping (No Phase Wrap).

IDEAL can be used available (see grab bag in spine section).

Sequence 1.5	TR	TE	ETL or FA	Band-width	F Matrix	Ph Matrix	FOV	Slice Thick	Inter-space	NEX	TI	Pulse Sequence Options

Table 3-6 Site Protocol: Routine Humerus

(Continued)

Table 3-6 Site Protocol: Routine Humerus—*cont'd*

Sequence 3T	TR	TE	ETL or FA	Band-width	F Matrix	Ph Matrix	FOV	Slice Thick	Inter-space	NEX	TI	Pulse Sequence Options

MRI OF THE ELBOW

Acquire three-plane pilot per site specifications.

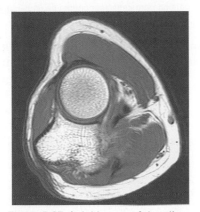

Figure 3-25 Axial image of the elbow

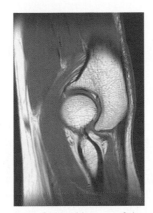

Figure 3-26 Sagittal image of the elbow

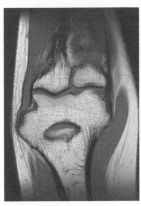

Figure 3-27 Coronal image of the elbow

COIL: Extremity coil or vendor-specific coil

POSITION: Prone, head first with affected arm extended. Place cushion under the patient's lower legs.

Off-center the patient to place the arm as close to isocenter as possible.

LANDMARK: Decubital fold or olecranon process

IMMOBILIZATION: Cushions around elbow with arm extended and pronated. Support the forearm and hand with cushions.

Acquisition of Axial Images of the Elbow

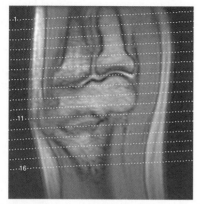

Figure 3-28 Coronal image of the elbow with axial locations

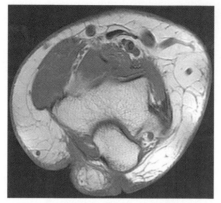

Figure 3-29 Axial image of the elbow

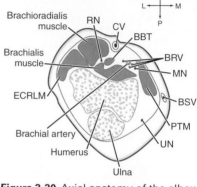

Figure 3-30 Axial anatomy of the elbow

KEY: **BBT**, biceps brachii tendon; **BSV**, basilic vein; **BRV**, brachial veins; **CV**, cephalic vein; **ECRLM**, extensor carpi radialis longus muscles; **MN**, medial nerve; **PTM**, pronator teres muscle; **RN**, radial nerve; **UN**, ulnar nerve.

SLICE ACQUISITION: Distal to proximal
SLICE ALIGNMENT: Parallel to the humeral condyles (trochlea and capitellum)
ANATOMICAL COVERAGE: Distal humerus through radial tuberosity

TIP: For bicep tendon tear, scan thorough radial tuberosity.

Acquisition of Coronal Images of the Elbow

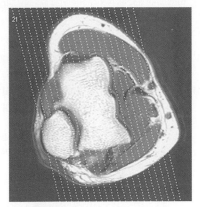

Figure 3-31 Axial image of the elbow with coronal locations

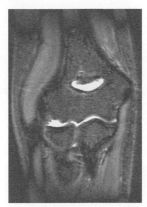

Figure 3-32 Coronal image of the elbow

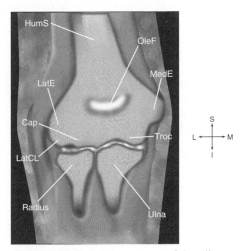

Figure 3-33 Coronal anatomy of the elbow

SLICE ACQUISITION: Anterior to posterior

SLICE ALIGNMENT: Parallel to medial and lateral epicondyle of the humerus

ANATOMIC COVERAGE: Include the margins of the skin and musculature, distal humerus to radial tuberosity.

TIP: Saturation (inferior) and saturation (superior) should be in the field of view to eliminate vascular motion.

KEY: **Cap**, capitulum; **HumS**, humeral shaft; **LatCL**, lateral condyle; **LatE**, lateral epicondyle; **MedE**, medial epicondyle; **OleF**, olecranon fossa; **Troc**, trochlea.

Acquisition of Sagittal Images of the Elbow

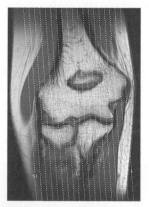

Figure 3-34 Coronal image of the elbow with sagittal locations

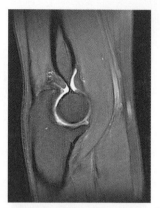

Figure 3-35 Sagittal image of the elbow

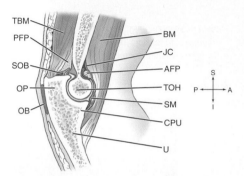

Figure 3-36 Sagittal anatomy of the elbow

SLICE ACQUISITION: Lateral to medial

SLICE ALIGNMENT: Parallel to the long axis of the humerus and forearm, perpendicular to the joint space

ANATOMIC COVERAGE: Include the margins of the skin and musculature, distal humerus to radial tuberosity

KEY: **AFP**, anterior fat pad; **BM**, brachialis muscle; **CPU**, coronoid process of ulna; **JC**, joint capsule; **SM**, synovial membrane; **OB**, olecranon bursa; **OP**, olecranon process; **PEP**, posterior fat pad; **SOB**, subtendinous olecranon bursa; **TBM**, triceps brachii muscle; **TOH**, trochlea of humerus; **U**, ulna.

TIP: Always reference axial image to ensure locs are perpendicular to the coronal plane.

Table 3-7 Routine Elbow

Sequence 1.5	TR	TE	ETL or FA	Band-width	F Matrix	Ph Matrix	FOV	Slice Thick	Inter-space	NEX	TI	Pulse Sequence Options
Ax PD FSE	3000	30	10	31.25	256	224	12-14	4	1	3		Sat S-I, FC
Ax T2 FS	3500	65	15	31.25	256	224	12-14	4	1	3		Sat S-I, F, FC
Cor FSE IR	3500	42	5	31.25	256	160	14/.80	3-4	0	2	110-150	Sat S-I, FC, seq
Cor T1 FSE	650	Min	3	31.25	256	224	14/.80	3-4	0	3		Sat S-I
Sag T2 FS	3500	65	15	31.25	256	224	14/14	3-4	0	3		Sat S-I, F, FC, NPW
OPT 3D SPGR C-+	Mach	Full	10FA	15.63	320	192	14	2.2	30locs/ slab	3		FSPGR, 3-D, Sat, Special, Zip 2, Zip 512

(Continued)

Table 3-7	Routine Elbow—*cont'd*											
Sequence 3T	**TR**	**TE**	**ETL or FA**	**Band-width**	**F Matrix**	**Ph Matrix**	**FOV**	**Slice Thick**	**Inter-space**	**NEX**	**TI**	**Pulse Sequence Options**
Ax PD FSE	3400	28	9	41.67	320	224	14/14	4	1	2		Sat S-I, FC
Ax T2 FS	3500	65	15	31.25	256	224	12-14	4	1	3		Sat S-I, F, FC
Cor IR FSE	3500	53	13	50	256	192	12/12	3	0	2	190	Sat S-I, FC, seq
Cor T1 FSE	1200	20	3	41.67	384	224	14/.80	3	0	2		Sat S-I
Sag T2 FS	4000	60	17	41.67	320	224	14/14	3	0	2		Sat S-I, F, FC
OPT Cor 3D GREC-+	Mach	Full	15FA	20	256	256	14/14	2	30 locs/ slab	2	51	FGRE, 3-D, Sat Special, Zip 2, Zip 512

FSE ETL 4 of lower.
TRF (Tailor Radio-Frequency) should be used with all FSE sequences to increase # of slices per TR.
Use NPW when possibility of anatomy wrapping (No Phase Wrap).
IDEAL can be used available (see grab bag in spine section).
Special is a 3D fat saturated technique.

Table 3-8 Site Protocol: Routine Elbow

Sequence 1.5	TR	TE	ETL or FA	Band-width	F Matrix	Ph Matrix	FOV	Slice Thick	Inter-space	NEX	TI	Pulse Sequence Options

Sequence 3T	TR	TE	ETL or FA	Band-width	F Matrix	Ph Matrix	FOV	Slice Thick	Inter-space	NEX	TI	Pulse Sequence Options

MRI OF THE FOREARM

Acquire three-plane pilot per site specifications.

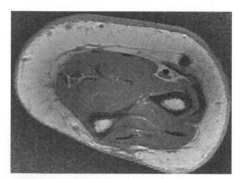

Figure 3-37 Axial image of the forearm

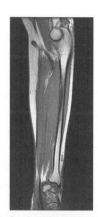

Figure 3-38 Sagittal image of the forearm

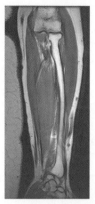

Figure 3-39 Coronal image of the forearm

COIL: Multi-channel torso coil, cardiac coil, or vendor-specific coil

POSITION: Swimmer's position, head first, body in anterior oblique position, arm extended forward. When patient size permits, or when wide bore is available, position arm at patient's side at isocenter.

LANDMARK: Midshaft of the forearm

IMMOBILIZATION: Sponges and Velcro straps to secure the forearm. Support the humerus and hand with sponges

Acquisition of Axial Images of the Forearm

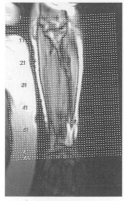

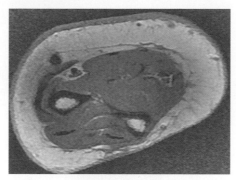

Figure 3-41 Axial image of the forearm

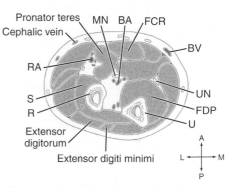

Figure 3-42 Axial anatomy of the forearm

Figure 3-40 Coronal image of the forearm with axial locations

SLICE ACQUISITION: Distal to proximal, wrist to elbow

SLICE ALIGNMENT: Perpendicular to the shaft of the ulna and radius

ANATOMIC COVERAGE: Proximal metacarpals to the distal humerus, including both joints

KEY: **BA**, brachialis artery; **BV**, basilic vein; **FCR**, flexor carpi radialis; **FDP**, flexor digitorum profundus; **MN**, median nerve; **R**, radius; **RA**, radial artery; **S**, supinator; **U**, ulna; **UN**, ulnar nerve.

Acquisition of Coronal Images of the Forearm

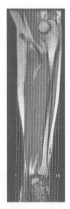

Figure 3-43 Sagittal image of the forearm with coronal locs

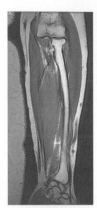

Figure 3-44 Coronal image of the forearm

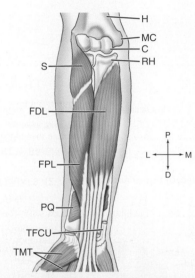

Figure 3-45 Coronal anatomy of forearm

SLICE ACQUISITION: Anterior to posterior

SLICE ALIGNMENT: Parallel to the shaft of the ulna or radius

ANATOMIC COVERAGE: Metacarpals to the distal humerus, including both the joints and musculature

KEY: C, capitellum; **FDL,** flexor digitorum profundus; **FPL,** flexor pollicis longus; **H,** humerus; **MC,** medial condyle; **RH,** radial head; **TMT,** thenar muscles of thumb; **TFCU,** tendon of flexor carpi ulnaris (cut); **PQ,** pronator quadratus; **S,** supinator.

Acquisition of Sagittal Images of the Forearm

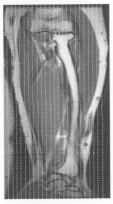

Figure 3-46 Coronal image of the forearm with sagittal locations

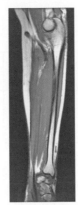

Figure 3-47 Sagittal image of the forearm

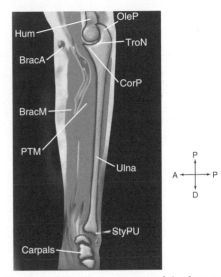

Figure 3-48 Sagittal anatomy of the forearm

SLICE ACQUISITION: Lateral to medial

SLICE ALIGNMENT: Parallel to shaft of ulna and radius

ANATOMIC COVERAGE: Metacarpals to distal humerus, including both joints and musculature.

KEY: **BracM**, brachialis muscle; **BracA**, brachial artery; **CorP**, coronoid process; **Hum**, humerus; **OleP**, olecranon process; **PTM**, pronator teres muscle; **StyPU**, styloid process of ulna; **TroN**, trochlear notch.

Table 3-9 Routine Forearm

Sequence 1.5	TR	TE	ETL or FA	Band-width	F Matrix	Ph Matrix	FOV	Slice Thick	Inter-space	NEX	TI	Pulse Sequence Options
Cor T1 FSE	500	Min	4	31.25	320	224	30/.75	3	1	3		Sat S-I, NPW
Cor IR FSE	4000	42	7	31.25	256	192	30/.75	3	1	3	150	Sat S-I, FC, seq, NPW
Ax PD FSE	3000	30	10	31.25	256	224	12-14	5	.5-1	3		Sat S-I, FC, NPW
Ax T2 FSE FS	3500	65	11	41.67	256	192	12-14	5	.5-1	3		Sat S-I, F, FC, TRF, NPW
Sag T2 FRFSE FS	4000	60	15	41.67	320	224	30/.75	3	0	2		Sat S-I, F, FC
OPT Sag FSE IR	4000	42		41.67	256	224	30/.75	3	0	2	190	Sat S-I, FC, Seq

Table 3-9 Routine Forearm—*cont'd*

Sequence 3T	TR	TE	ETL or FA	Band-width	F Matrix	Ph Matrix	FOV	Slice Thick	Inter-space	NEX	TI	Pulse Sequence Options
Cor T1 FSE	1200	20	3	41.67	384	224	30/.75	3	0	2		Sat S-I, NPW
Cor IR FSE	4000	42	25	41.67	256	192	30/.75	3	0	2	190	Sat S-I, FC, seq, NPW
Ax PD FSE	3000	30	10	31.25	256	224	12-14	5	.5-1	3		Sat S-I, FC, NPW
Ax T2 FS	3500	65	15	50	320	224	15/15	5	.5-1	2		Sat S-I, FC, NPW
Sag T2 FRFSE FS	4000	60	15	41.67	320	224	30/.75	3	0	2		Sat S-I, F, FC
OPT Sag FSE IR	4000	42		41.67	256	224	30/.75	3	0	2	190	Sat S-I, FC, seq
Cor T1 FSE	1200	20	3	41.67	384	224	30/.75	3	0	2		Sat S-I, NPW
Cor IR FSE	4000	42	25	41.67	256	192	30/.75	3	0	2	190	Sat S-I, FC, Seq, NPW

FSE ETL 4 of lower.
TRF (Tailor Radio-Frequency) should be used with all FSE sequences to increase # of slices per TR.
Use NPW when possibility of anatomy wrapping (No Phase Wrap).
IDEAL can be used available (see grab bag in spine section).

Table 3-10 Site Protocol: Routine Forearm

Sequence 1.5	TR	TE	ETL or FA	Band-width	F Matrix	Ph Matrix	FOV	Slice Thick	Inter-space	NEX	TI	Pulse Sequence Options

Table 3-10	Site Protocol: Routine Forearm—cont'd												
Sequence 3T	TR	TE	ETL or FA	Band-width	F Matrix	Ph Matrix	FOV	Slice Thick	Inter-space	NEX	TI	Pulse Sequence Options

MRI OF THE WRIST

Acquire three-plane pilot per site specifications.

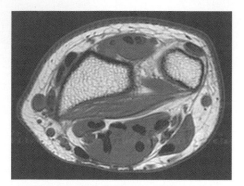

Figure 3-49 Axial image of the wrist

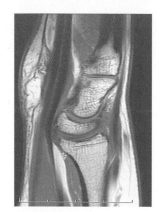

Figure 3-50 Sagittal image of the wrist

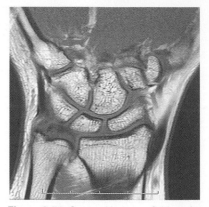

Figure 3-51 Coronal image of the wrist

COIL: Multi-channel vendor-specific wrist coil or extremity coil

POSITION: When patient size permits, or when wide bore is available, position wrist at isocenter Swimmer's position, head first, body in anterior oblique position, arm extended forward

LANDMARK: Midcarpals, ulnar styloid process

IMMOBILIZATION: Use sponges and Velcro straps to secure the hand and wrist, and support forearm and humerus. Place long-angle sponge under patient's torso.

TIP: Patient comfort is key to maintain accurate positioning throughout scan.

Acquisition of Coronal Images of the Wrist

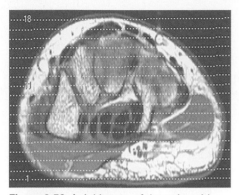

Figure 3-52 Axial image of the wrist with coronal locations

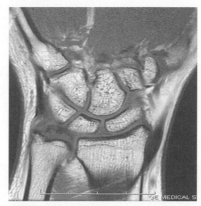

Figure 3-53 Coronal image of the wrist

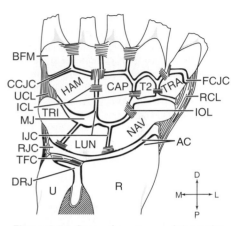

Figure 3-54 Coronal anatomy of the wrist

SLICE ACQUISITION: Anterior to posterior
SLICE ALIGNMENT: Parallel to carpal tunnel, pisiform to scaphoid
ANATOMIC COVERAGE: Proximal metacarpals to the distal ulna and radius; include all musculature

TIP: Place saturation (inferior) band proximal to the metacarpals to reduce vascular motion.

KEY: **AC**, articular ligament; **BFM**, base of fifth metacarpal; **CCJC**, common carpometacarpal joint and compartment; **DRJ**, distal radioulnar joint; **FCJC**, first carpometacarpal joint compartment; **ICL**, intercarpal ligaments; **IJC**, intercarpal joints and compartment; **IOL**, interosseous ligament; **MJ**, midcarpal joint (mediocarpal compartment); **R**, radius; **RCL**, radial collateral ligament; **RJC**, radiocarpal joint and compartment; **TFC**, triangular tibrocartilage complex (articular disk); **U**, ulna; **UCL**, ulnar collateral ligament.

Acquisition of Axial Images of the Wrist

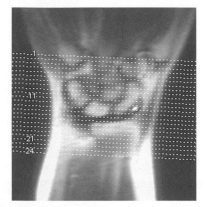

Figure 3-55 Coronal image of the wrist with axial locations

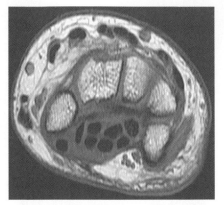

Figure 3-56 Axial image of the wrist

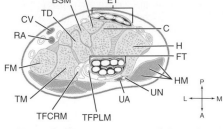

Figure 3-57 Axial anatomy of the wrist

SLICE ACQUISITION: Distal to proximal
SLICE ALIGNMENT: Perpendicular to the shaft of the ulna and radius
ANATOMIC COVERAGE: Proximal metacarpals to distal ulna and radius

KEY: BTM, base of third metacarpal; **BSM,** base of second metacarpal; **C,** capitate; **CV,** cephalic vein; **ET,** extensor tendons; **FM,** first metacarpal; **FT,** flexor tendons; **H,** hamate; **HM,** hypothenar muscles; **RA,** radial artery; **TD,** trapezoid; **TFCRM,** tendon of flexor carpi radialis muscle; **TFPLM,** tendon of flexor pollicis longus muscle; **TM,** trapezium; **UA,** ulnar artery; **UN,** ulnar nerve.

Acquisition of Sagittal Images of the Wrist

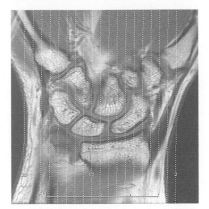

Figure 3-58 Coronal image of the wrist with sagittal locations

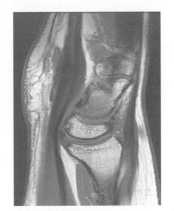

Figure 3-59 Sagittal image of the wrist

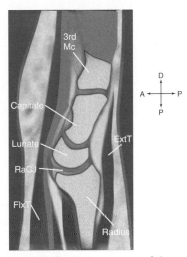

Figure 3-60 Sagittal anatomy of the wrist

SLICE ACQUISITION: Lateral to medial

SLICE ALIGNMENT: Parallel to the metacarpals and phalanges

ANATOMIC COVERAGE: Thumb through the fifth digit, including the distal ulna and radius, palmar to the dorsal surface

TIP: Place the inferior saturation band proximal to the carpals to reduce vascular motion.

KEY: **3rdMc**, 3rd metacarpal; **ExtT**, extensor tendons; **FlxT**, flexo tendons; **RaCJ**, radialcarpal joint.

Table 3-11   Routine Wrist

Sequence 1.5	TR	TE	ETL or FA	Band-width	F Matrix	Ph Matrix	FOV	Slice Thick	Inter-space	NEX	TI	Pulse Sequence Options
Cor 3-D FSPGR		Full	10FA	15.63	320	192	10-12	2.0	30locs/ slab	3		3-D, Sat, Special, Zip 2, Zip 512
Cor PD FSE FS	3500	20	11	31.25	320	224	10-12	3	0	4		Sat S-I, Fat, FC
Cor T1 FSE	700	Min	4	31.25	448	256	10-12	3	0	3		Sat S-I
Ax PD FRFSE FS	3000	30	9	41.67	320	256	10-12	3	.5	4		Sat S-I, Fat, FC
Sag PD FRFSE FS	3500	40	9	41.67	288	256	12-14	3	0	2		Sat S-I, Fat, FC, NPW
OPT 3D SPGR C-+	Mach	Full	10FA	15.63	320	192	12/12	2.2	30locs/ slab	3		FSPGR, 3D, Sat, Special, Zip 2, Zip 512

Table 3-11 Routine Wrist—*cont'd*

Sequence 3T	TR	TE	ETL or FA	Band-width	F Matrix	Ph Matrix	FOV	Slice Thick	Inter-space	NEX	TI	Pulse Sequence Options
Cor 3D GRE	Mach	Full	15FA	20	256	256	8/8	1.8	20 locs/ slab	2	51	GRE, 3-D, Sat, Special, Zip 2, Zip 512, Fast
Cor PD FSE FS	2000	42	11	41.67	448	224	10/10	2.5	0	4		FSE-XL, Sat S-I, Fat, FC, TRF
Cor T1 FSE	900	Min	4	41.67	448	256	10/10	2.5	0	2		FSE-XL, Sat S-I, TRF
Ax PD FRFSE FS	3500	30	9	41.67	320	224	10-12	3	1	4		FRFSE, Sat S-I, Fat, FC, TRF, NPW
Sag PD FRFSE FS	3500	40	9	50	288	256	12/12	2.5	0	2		FRFSE, Sat S-I, Fat, FC, TRF, NPW
OPT Cor 3D FGRE C-+	Mach	Full	15FA	20	256	256	12/12	2	30 locs/ slab	2	51	FGRE, 3D, Sat, Special, Zip 2, Zip 512

FSE ETL 4 of lower.
TRF (Tailor Radio-Frequency) should be used with all FSE sequences to increase # of slices per TR.
Use NPW when possibility of anatomy wrapping (No Phase Wrap).
IDEAL can be used available (see grab bag in spine).
Use OPT SPGR and GRE for C-+ when indicate.

Table 3-12   Site Protocol: Routine Wrist

Sequence 1.5	TR	TE	ETL or FA	Band-width	F Matrix	Ph Matrix	FOV	Slice Thick	Inter-space	NEX	TI	Pulse Sequence Options

Sequence 3T	TR	TE	ETL or FA	Band-width	F Matrix	Ph Matrix	FOV	Slice Thick	Inter-space	NEX	TI	Pulse Sequence Options

MRI OF THE HAND AND DIGITS

Acquire three-plane pilot per site specifications.

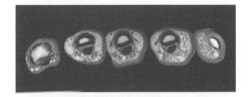

Figure 3-61 Axial image of the hand

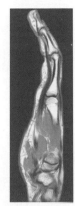

Figure 3-62 Sagittal image of the hand

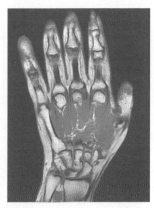

Figure 3-63 Coronal image of the hand

COIL: Multi-channel vendor-specific hand coil or extremity coil

POSITION: Swimmer's position, head first, body in anterior oblique position, arm extended forward. When patient size permits, or when wide bore is available, position hand at isocenter.

Hand in coil with the fingers extended and immobilized

LANDMARK: Distal metacarpals

IMMOBILIZATION: Support the forearm and humerus with sponges. Place long-angle sponge under the patient's torso.

TIP: For digits, follow the same protocol using a smaller field of view.

Acquisition of Coronal Images of the Hand

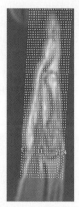

Figure 3-64 Sagittal image of the hand with coronal locations

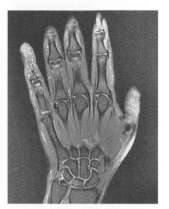

Figure 3-65 Coronal image of the hand

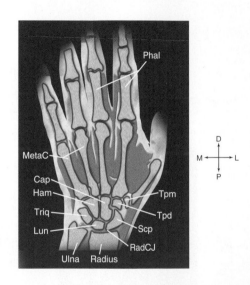

Figure 3-66 Coronal anatomy of the hand

SLICE ACQUISITION: Anterior to posterior
SLICE ALIGNMENT: Perpendicular to the digits and metacarpals
ANATOMIC COVERAGE: Thumb through the fifth digit, distal phalanx to the styloid process of the ulna
Cross-reference the sagittal pilot.

TIP: Reference the three-plane pilot to ensure proper coverage.
Place the saturation (inferior) band proximal to the carpals to reduce vascular motion.

KEY: **Cap**, capitate; **Ham**, hamate; **Lun**, lunate; **MetaC**, metacarpals; **Phal**, phalanx; **RadCJ**, radialcarpal joint; **Scp**, scaphoid; **Tpm**, trapezium; **Tpd**, trapezoid; **Triq**, triquetrum.

Acquisition of Axial Images of the Hand

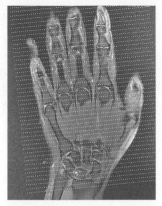

Figure 3-67 Coronal image of the hand with axial locations

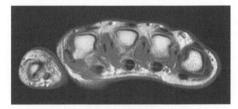

Figure 3-68 Axial image of the hand

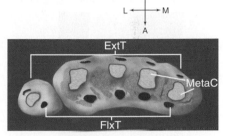

Figure 3-69 Axial anatomy of the hand

SLICE ACQUISITION: Distal to proximal
SLICE ALIGNMENT: Perpendicular to the digits and metacarpals
ANATOMIC COVERAGE: Distal phalanx to the styloid process of the ulna

TIP: Reference the three-plane pilot to ensure proper coverage.

KEY: **ExtT**, extensor tendons; **FlxT**, flexor tendons; **MetaC**, metacarpals.

191

Acquisition of Sagittal Images of the Hand

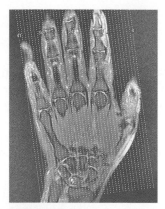

Figure 3-70 Coronal image of the hand with sagittal locations

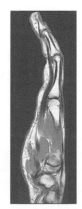

Figure 3-71 Sagittal image of the hand

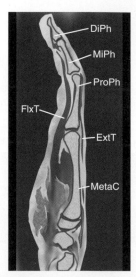

Figure 3-72 Sagittal anatomy of the hand

SLICE ACQUISITION: Lateral to medial

SLICE ALIGNMENT: Parallel to the digits and metacarpals

ANATOMIC COVERAGE: Thumb through the fifth digit, distal phalanx to the styloid process of the ulna

KEY: **DiPh**, distal phalanx; **ExtT**, extensor tendons; **FlxT**, flexor tendons; **MiPh**, middle phalanx; **MetaC**, metacarpals; **ProPh**, proximal phalanx.

> *TIP:* Reference the three-plane pilot to ensure proper coverage.
>
> Place the saturation (inferior) band proximal to the metacarpals to reduce vascular motion.

Table 3-13 Routine Hand

Sequence 1.5	TR	TE	ETL or FA	Band-width	F Matrix	Ph Matrix	FOV	Slice Thick	Inter-space	NEX	TI	Pulse Sequence Options
Cor T1 FSE	600	Min	4	31.25	384	224	20-24	2.5	0	4		Sat S-I
Cor IR FSE	3500	30	15	31.25	256	224	20-24	3.0	0	3	150	Sat S-I, TRF, seq
Ax PD FRFSE FS	3400	25	7	41.67	384	256	12-14	3.5	0	3		Sat S-I, F, FC, NPW
Ax T1 FSE	500	Min	4	31.25	384	224	12-14	3.5	0	3		Sat S-I, NPW
Sag PD FRFSE FS	2200	34	7	41.67	288	256	20-24	3.0	0	3		Sat S-I, F, FC, NPW
OPT Sag T1 FSE	600	Min	4	31.25	384	224	20-24	3.0	0	4		Sat S-I

(Continued)

| Table 3-13 | Routine Hand—*cont'd* |

Sequence 3T	TR	TE	ETL or FA	Band-width	F Matrix	Ph Matrix	FOV	Slice Thick	Inter-space	NEX	TI	Pulse Sequence Options
Cor T1 FSE	900	Min	4	41.67	448	256	20-24	2.5	0	2		Sat S-I
Cor IR FSE	4000	42	19	50	256	192	20-24	3.0	0	2	190	Sat S-I, FC, seq
Ax PD FRFSE FS	2000	32	9	50	320	224	12-14	3.5	1	3		Sat S-I, Fat, FC
Ax T1 FSE	1250	20	2	41.67	384	224	12-14	3.5	0	2		Sat S-I
Sag PD FRFSE FS	3000	20	9	50	288	256	20-24	2.5	0	3		Sat S-I, Fat, FC, NPW
OPT Sag T1 FSE	900	Min	4	41.67	448	256	20-24	2.5	0	2		Sat S-I, NPW

FSE ETL 4 of lower.

TRF (Tailor Radio-Frequency) should be used with all FSE sequences to increase # of slices per TR.

Use NPW when possibility of anatomy wrapping (No Phase Wrap).

IDEAL can be used available (see grab bag in spine).

Table 3-14 Site Protocol: Routine Hand

Sequence 1.5	TR	TE	ETL or FA	Band-width	F Matrix	Ph Matrix	FOV	Slice Thick	Inter-space	NEX	TI	Pulse Sequence Options

(Continued)

Table 3-14 Site Protocol: Routine Hand—*cont'd*

Sequence 3T	TR	TE	ETL or FA	Band-width	F Matrix	Ph Matrix	FOV	Slice Thick	Inter-space	NEX	TI	Pulse Sequence Options

MRI of the Lower Extremities

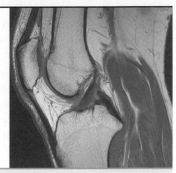

CHAPTER OUTLINE

MRI OF THE LOWER EXTREMITIES—CONSIDERATIONS

Scan Considerations

- Extremities should be scanned in the anatomical position when possible. Consider the patients tolerance for pain; a neutral position may be necessary.
- When scanning long bones, it may be difficult to fit the anatomy into a single coil. Repositioning the patient may be required.
- Place a vitamin E, capsule or MRI-compatible market at the area of pain or interest.
- Refer to all safety-related parameters.
- As the SAR (specific absorption rate) increases, the patient's body temperature will also increase. SAR elevation can be compensated for by increasing the TR slightly. If this is not done correctly at 3T, the SAR will increase and scanner will stop as a patient safety precaution. All 3T systems have SAR monitors that should be referenced while scanning. This is not an issue at 1.5T.
- Contrast is often used for osteomyelitis, tumor, or infection.
- MR arthrogram is performed to best demonstrate labral and intra-articular pathology of the hip. A mixture of gadolinium and iodinated contrast is injected into the bursa in a fluoroscopy suite before the MRI is performed. Indirect arthrography can be performed after injecting gadolinium into a vein and waiting a period of time while exercising the affected joint.

- Orthopedic hardware can cause distortion and metallic artifacts in the image. To help compensate, the bandwidth should be increased, the ETL can be increased, and the NEX (number of excitations) can be increased. These options will help but not eliminate these artifacts.

Coils

- Multi-channel body-specific coils are used when available. Any coil that covers the anatomy may be used, i.e., the cardiac coil may be used to scan the hip.
- All multi-channel coils produce excessive single adjacent to the coil. This can be compensated for by using vendor-specific options to provide uniform single intensity.

Pulse Sequences

- T1 is used to best identify anatomic structures, whereas T2 fat saturation (FS) and or STIR (short T1 inversion recovery) provides detailed evidence of pathology.
- On T1 sequences, bones should appear bright or hyperintense because fat in the bone has a short relaxation time. If not, a disease process can be present. On T1 Sequences, fluid will appear dark or hyperintense because water has a long T1 relaxation time.
- On T2 sequences, fluid produces bright or hyperintense signal as a result of long T2 relaxation. T2 imaging uses FS or

STIR to eliminate the fat and enhance abnormal fluid or pathology in bone.

- T1 FS is used post routine arthrogram to best visualize the contrast in the joints. T2 FS may also be added when indicated.
- T1 and/or T2 CUBE can be used to obtain high-resolution submillimeter images of the ankle.

Options

- FS options and terminology are vendor-specific. For GE system, use "fat classic" for FS with enhanced anatomical detail.
- IDEAL (GE) is a fat/water separation technique (previously called 3-point Dixon technique). This technique eliminates fat and water and provides an in and out of phase image, all in one acquisition. IDEAL can be used with T1, T2, and SPGR pulse sequences.
- Superior and inferior saturation bands help to compensate for vascular pulsation, whereas left or right saturation bands can help compensate for breathing or cardiac motion. Saturation bands can be used on all pulse sequences.
- Flow compensation (FC) or gradient nulling should be used on T2 images to help compensate for vascular motion.

MRI OF THE HIPS

Acquire three-plane pilot per site specifications.

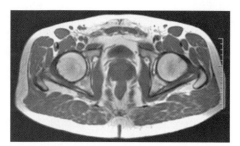

Figure 4-1 Axial image of the hips

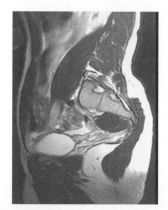

Figure 4-2 Sagittal image of the hip

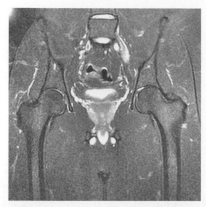

Figure 4-3 Coronal image of the hip

COIL: Multi-channel vendor-specific torso coil or cardiac coil
POSITION: Supine, feet first, legs flat and extended with feet inverted
LANDMARK: Pubic symphysis
IMMOBILIZATION: Place cushion between the ankles to support inversion of feet. Secure feet with tape.

TIP: FOV is dependent on patient size.

Acquisition of Axial Image of the Hips

Hips are scanned bilaterally in the axial and coronal plane; sagittal sequences are unilateral.

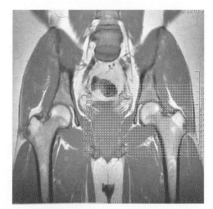

Figure 4-4 Coronal image of the hips with axial locations

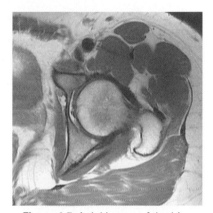

Figure 4-5 Axial image of the hips

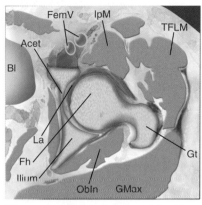

Figure 4-6 Axial anatomy of the hips

SLICE ACQUISITION: Superior to inferior

SLICE ALIGNMENT: Parallel to the femoral heads

ANATOMIC COVERAGE: Iliac fossa to proximal femur, including the lesser trochanter

TIP: Axial images may be done unilaterally when ordered by the physician.

KEY: **Acet**, acetebellum; **BI**, bladder; **FemV**, femoral vessels; **Fh**, femoral head; **Gt**, ; **Gmax**, gluteus maximus; **IpM**, iliopsoas muscle; **La**, ; **Obin**, obturator internus tendon; **TFLM**, tensor fascial latae muscle.

Acquisition of Coronal Image of the Hips

Hips are scanned bilaterally in the axial and coronal plane, and sagittal sequences are unilateral.

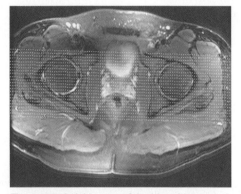

Figure 4-7 Axial image of the hip with coronal locations

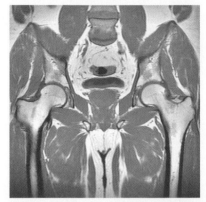

Figure 4-8 Coronal image of the hip: unilateral

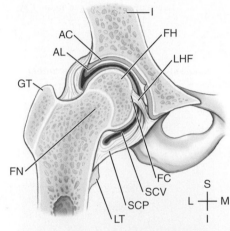

Figure 4-9 Coronal anatomy of the hips

SLICE ACQUISITION: Anterior to posterior
SLICE ALIGNMENT: Parallel to femoral heads
ANATOMIC COVERAGE: Pubis to posterior ischium

TIP: Coronal images may be done unilaterally when ordered by the physician.

KEY: **AC**, articular cartilage; **AL**, acetabular labrum; **FC**, fovea capitis; **FH**, femoral head; **FN**, femoral neck; **GT**, greater trochanter; **I**, illium; **LHF**, ligament of the head of the femur (ligamentum teres); **LT**, lesser trochanter; **SCP**, synovial capsule; **SCV**, synovial cavity.

Acquisition of Sagittal Image of the Hips

Hips are scanned bilaterally in the axial and coronal plane, and sagittal sequences are unilateral of the affected side.

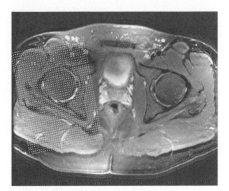

Figure 4-10 Axial image with sagittal locations

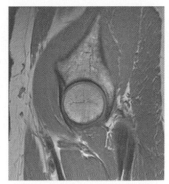

Figure 4-11 Sagittal image of the hip

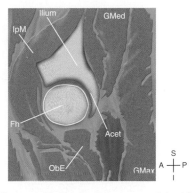

Figure 4-12 Sagittal anatomy of the hips

SLICE ACQUISITION: Lateral to medial
SLICE ALIGNMENT: Parallel to the labrum of the acetabulum
ANATOMIC COVERAGE: Greater trochanter to the superior pubic ramus

TIP: Sagittal images may also be prescribed off a coronal image. Use three-plane pilot to reference FOV.

Table 4-1 Routine Hip

Sequence 1.5	TR	TE	ETL or FA	Band-width	F Matrix	Ph Matrix	FOV	Slice Thick	Inter-space	NEX	TI	Pulse Sequence Options
Ax T2 FRFSE FS	3400	60	13	41.67	256	224	36-40	4	0	2		Sat S-I, F, FC, NPW
Ax T1 FSE	525	Min	4	31.25	384	224	36-40	4	0	2		Sat S-I, NPW
Cor T2 FRFSE FS	3400	60	11	41.67	256	224	36-40	4	0	2		Sat S-I, FC, NPW
Cor T1 FSE	350	Min	4	31.25	320	224	36-40	4	0	2		Sat S-I, NPW
Sag T2 FRFSE FS	3400	60	23	41.67	320	224	24/24	4	0	4		Sat, F-S-I, FC
OPT Ax PD FS	3500	20	7	50	320	224	16-18	4	.5	2		Sat S-I, NPW

Table 4-1												Routine Hip—cont'd
Sequence 3T	TR	TE	ETL or FA	Band-width	F Matrix	Ph Matrix	FOV	Slice Thick	Inter-space	NEX	TI	Pulse Sequence Options
Ax T2 FRFSE FS	4550	68	25	50	448	224	34-38	3	.3	2		Sat S-I-F, FC
Ax T1 FSE	800	Min	4	50	512	224	34-38	3	.3	2		Sat S-I
Cor T2 FRFSE FS	3300	68	25	50	448	224	32/32	3	.3	2		Sat S-I, FC, NPW
Cor T1 FSE	1200	Min	2	50	512	224	32/32	3	.3	2		Sat S-I, NPW
Sag T2 FRFSE FS	3200	68	27	50	448	224	22/22	3.5	0	3		Sat S-I-F, FC, NPW
OPT Ax PD	3500	30	7	50	320	224	14-16	3	.3	2		Sat S-I, NPW

T1 FSE ETL 4 of lower.

Sagittal images are done of affected side.

Reduce FOV and increase the NEX when axial images are ordered on the affected side only

TRF (Tailor Radio-Frequency) should be used with all FSE sequences to increase # of slices per TR.

Use NPW when possibility of anatomy wrapping (No Phase Wrap)

Coronal STIR can be used when there is incomplete FS. Use unilateral Axial PD for labral pathology

IDEAL can be used available (see grab bag in spine section)

Table 4-2 Site Protocol: Routine Hip

Sequence 1.5	TR	TE	ETL or FA	Band-width	F Matrix	Ph Matrix	FOV	Slice Thick	Inter-space	NEX	TI	Pulse Sequence Options

Table 4-2	Site Protocol: Routine Hip—*cont'd*												
Sequence 3T	TR	TE	ETL or FA	Band-width	F Matrix	Ph Matrix	FOV	Slice Thick	Inter-space	NEX	TI	Pulse Sequence Options

MRI OF THE FEMUR

Acquire three-plane pilot per site specifications.

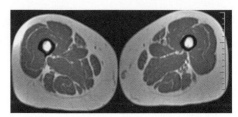

Figure 4-13 Axial image of the femur

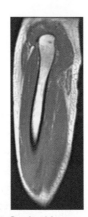

Figure 4-14 Sagittal image of the femur

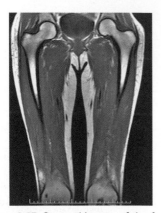

Figure 4-15 Coronal image of the femur

COIL: Vendor-specific eight-channel torso coil or cardiac coil.
POSITION: Supine, feet first, legs flat and extended with feet inverted.
LANDMARK: Midshaft of the femur
IMMOBILIZATION: Place a cushion between the ankles to support inversion of feet. Secure patient's feet with tape.

TIP: Use long-bone protocol. FOV is determined by the anatomy to be covered.
 If off center, the FOV diminishes adequate fat saturation; STIR should be performed.

Acquisition of Coronal Image of the Femur

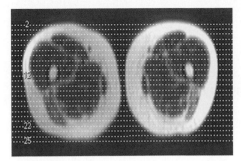

Figure 4-16 Axial image of the femurs with bilateral coronal locations

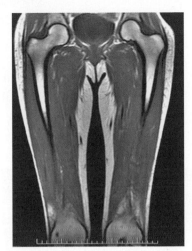

Figure 4-17 Coronal image of the femur

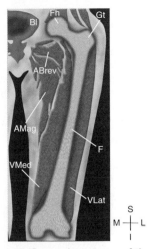

Figure 4-18 Coronal anatomy of the femur

SLICE ACQUISITION: Anterior to posterior

SLICE ALIGNMENT: Parallel to the shaft of the femur

ANATOMICAL COVERAGE: Head of femur to proximal tibia; include musculature of the thigh.

KEY: **ABrev**, adductor brevis muscle; **AMag**, adductor magnus muscle; **Bl**, bladder; **F**, femur; **Fh**, femoral head; **Gt**, greater trochanter; **VLat**, vastus lateralis muscle; **VMed**, vastus medialis muscle.

TIP: Reference sagittal image of pilot for superior to inferior anatomic coverage. Coronal plane scanned bilaterally for comparison.

Acquisition of Axial Image of the Femur

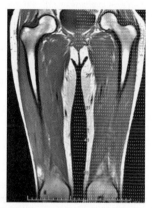

Figure 4-19 Coronal image of the femur with unilateral axial locations

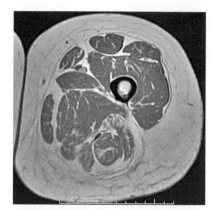

Figure 4-20 Axial image of the femur

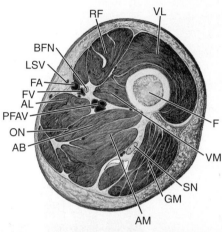

Figure 4-21 Axial anatomy of the femur

SLICE ACQUISITION: Superior to inferior
SLICE ALIGNMENT: Perpendicular to the shaft of the femur
ANATOMIC COVERAGE: From the head of the femur to the tibial plateau

KEY: **AB**, adductor brevis; **AL**, adductor longus; **AM**, adductor magnus; **BFN**, branches of femoral nerve; **F**, femur; **FA**, femoral artery; **FV**, femoral vein; **GM**, gluteus maximus; **LSV**, long saphenous vein; **ON**, obturator nerve; **PFAV**, profundus femoris artery and veins; **RF**, rectus femoris; **SN**, sciatic nerve; **VL**, vastus lateralis; **VM**, vastus medialis.

Acquisition of Sagittal Image of the Femur

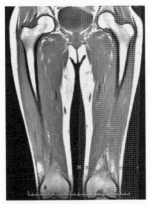

Figure 4-22 Coronal image of the femur with unilateral sagittal locations

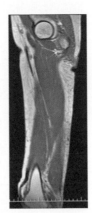

Figure 4-23 Sagittal image of the femur

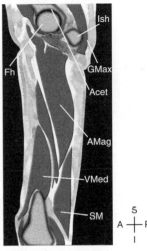

Figure 4-24 Sagittal anatomy of the femur

SLICE ACQUISITION: Lateral to medial

SLICE ALIGNMENT: Parallel to the shaft of the femur

ANATOMIC COVERAGE: Greater trochanter and lateral condyle to the femoral head and medial condyle, head of the femur to the tibial plateau; include musculature of the thigh.

KEY: **Acet**, acetebellum; **AMag**, adductor magnus muscle; **Fh**, femoral head; **GMax**, gluteus maximus; **Ish**, ischium; **SM**, semimembranosus muscle; **VMed**, vastus medials muscle.

| Table 4-3 | Routine Femurs: Long Bone Protocol |

Sequence 1.5	TR	TE	ETL or FA	Band-width	F Matrix	Ph Matrix	FOV	Slice Thick	Inter-space	NEX	TI	Pulse Sequence Options
Cor STIR	3500	42	5	31.25	256	160	38-46	4.0	1.0	3	110-150	Sat, S-I, FC, Seq
Cor T1 FSE	450	Min	4	31.25	320	224	38-46	4.0	1.0	2		Sat S-I
Ax. STIR	3000	40	7	41.67	256	192	32-46	4.0	1.5	3	150	Sat, S-I, FC, Seq
Ax.T1 FSE	600	Min	3-4	31.25	256	224	32-46	4.0	1.5	2		Sat S-I
OPT Sag STIR	3500	40	7	41.67	256	192	38-46	4.0	1.0	3	150	Sat, S-I, FC, Seq
Post GAD												
Cor T1 FSE FS	625	Min	3	41.67	256	224	26-28	4	0	3		FSE-XL, Sat F, A, TRF, NPW
Ax.T1 FSE FS	450	14	4	35.71	256	224	26-28	3	1	3		FSE-XL, Sat A, Fat, TRF, NPW

Table 4-3				Routine Femurs: Long Bone Protocol—*cont'd*								
Sequence 3T	**TR**	**TE**	**ETL or FA**	**Band-width**	**F Matrix**	**Ph Matrix**	**FOV**	**Slice Thick**	**Inter-space**	**NEX**	**TI**	**Pulse Sequence Options**
Cor STIR	3500	50	13	50	256	192	38-46	4.0	1.0	2	180-200	Sat S-I, FC, Seq
Cor T1 FSE	900	Min	4	50	448	224	38-46	4	.4	1		Sat S-I
Ax. STIR	3500	50	13	50	256	192	32-46	4.0	1.0	2	180-200	Sat S-I, FC, Seq
Ax.T1 FSE	1100	Min	4	50	448	224	32-46	5	0	1		Sat S-I
OPT Sag STIR	3500	50	11	50	448	224	38-46	4	0	2		Sat S-I, FC, Seq
Post GAD												
Cor T1 FS	900	Min	4	50	448	224	24-26	4	1	2		Sat S-I, F, NPW
Ax.T1 FS	1100	Min	4	50	448	224	24-26	4	1.5	2		Sat S-I, F, NPW

T1 FSE ETL 4 of lower.

When contrast is indicated perform unilateral sequences on affected side.

TRF (Tailor Radio-Frequency) should be used with all FSE sequences to increase # of slices per TR.

Use NPW when possibility of anatomy wrapping (No Phase Wrap)

IDEAL can be used available (see grab bag in spine section)

| Table 4-4 | | | Site Protocol: Long Bone Protocol | | | | | | | | | | |

Sequence 1.5	TR	TE	ETL or FA	Band-width	F Matrix	Ph Matrix	FOV	Slice Thick	Inter-space	NEX	TI	Pulse Sequence Options
Post GAD												

Sequence 3T	TR	TE	ETL or FA	Band-width	F Matrix	Ph Matrix	FOV	Slice Thick	Inter-space	NEX	TI	Pulse Sequence Options
Post GAD												

Table 4-4 Site Protocol: Long Bone Protocol—*cont'd*

MRI OF THE KNEE

Acquire three-plane pilot per site specifications.

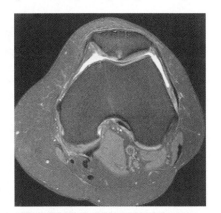 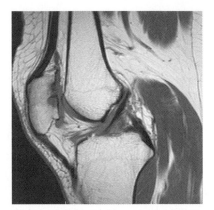 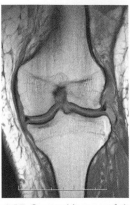

Figure 4-25 Axial image of the knee   **Figure 4-26** Sagittal image of the knee   **Figure 4-27** Coronal image of the knee

COIL: Multi-channel vendor-specific knee coil

POSITION: Supine, feet first, with knee positioned in the coil as close to the isocenter as possible

LANDMARK: Apex of the patella

IMMOBILIZATION: Surround the knee with sponges, cushion under heel, and support the lower leg and ankle.

Acquisition of Axial Image of the Knee

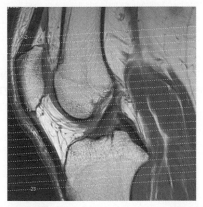

Figure 4-28 Sagittal image of the knee with axial locs

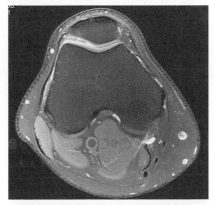

Figure 4-29 Axial image of the knee

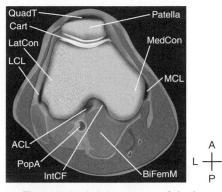

Figure 4-30 Axial anatomy of the knee

KEY: ACL, anterior cruciate ligament; **BiFemM**, biceps femoris muscle; **Cart**, cartilage; **IntCF**, intercondylar fossa; **LatCon**, lateral condyle; **LCL**, lateral collateral ligament; **MedCon**, medial condyle; **MCL**, medial collateral ligament; **PopA**, popliteal artery; **QuadT**, quadricep tendon.

SLICE ACQUISITION: Superior to inferior
SLICE ALIGNMENT: Parallel to the tibial platcau
ANATOMIC COVERAGE: From above the patella through the tibial tuberosity and the patella tendon insertion

TIP: Axial sequences may be plotted on either sagittal or coronal images.
Reference the three-plane pilot to ensure correct alignment and adequate anatomic coverage.

Acquisition of Sagittal Image of the Knee

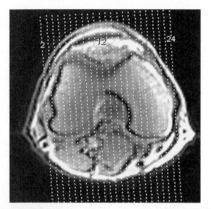

Figure 4-31 Coronal image of the knee with sagittal locations

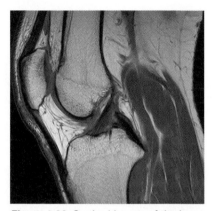

Figure 4-32 Sagittal image of the knee

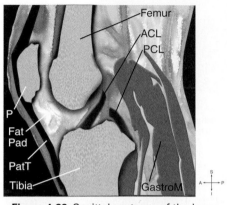

Figure 4-33 Sagittal anatomy of the knee

KEY: ACL, anterior cruciate ligament; **P**, patella; **PatT**, patellar tendon; **PCL**, posterior cruciate ligament.

SLICE ACQUISITION: Medial to lateral

SLICE ALIGNMENT: Parallel to the anterior cruciate ligament

ANATOMIC COVERAGE: From the medial condyle of the femur to the lateral condyle of the femur

TIP: Coronal image must be referenced on three-plane pilot to ensure superior to inferior coverage. Saturation (superior) and (inferior) in the field of view to reduce vascular motion.

Acquisition of Coronal Image of the Knee

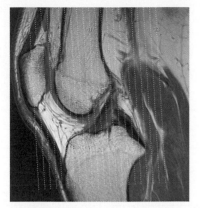

Figure 4-34 Sagittal image of the knee with coronal locations

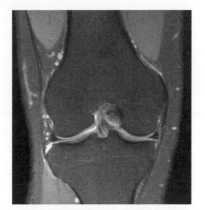

Figure 4-35 Coronal image of the knee

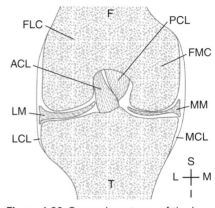

Figure 4-36 Coronal anatomy of the knee

SLICE ACQUISITION: Anterior to posterior
SLICE ALIGNMENT: Parallel to the posterior margins of the femoral condyles
ANATOMIC COVERAGE: From the patella through the femoral condyles

KEY: **ACL**, anterior cruciate ligament; **F**, femur; **FLC**, femur, lateral condyle; **FMC**, femur medial condyle; **LCL**, lateral collateral ligament; **LM**, lateral meniscus; **MCL**, medial lateral ligament; **MM**, medial meniscus; **PCL**, posterior cruciate ligament; **T**, tibia.

TIP: When plotting off a sagittal image, always reference the axial to ensure slices are parallel to the femoral condyles. Always reference the three-plane pilot to ensure correct alignment and adequate anatomic coverage. Saturation (superior) and (inferior) in the FOV to reduce vascular motion.

Table 4-5 Routine Knee

Sequence 1.5	TR	TE	ETL or FA	Band-width	F Matrix	Ph Matrix	FOV	Slice Thick	Inter-space	NEX	TI	Pulse Sequence Options
Sag PD FRFSE FS	3000	34	7	41.67	320	224	14/14	3.5	0	2		Sat S-I, F, FC, NPW
Sag T1 FSE	600	Min	4	41.67	512	192	14/14	3.5	0	2		Sat S-I, NPW
Ax PD FRFSE FS	2100	20	7	41.67	512	224	14/14	3.5	1	2		Sat S-I, F, FC, NPW
Cor PD-T2 FSE FS	3000	20/ 80	10	41.67	320	224	14/14	3.5	.5	2		Sat S-I, F, FC, NPW

Table 4-5	Routine Knee—*cont'd*											
Sequence 3T	**TR**	**TE**	**ETL or FA**	**Band-width**	**F Matrix**	**Ph Matrix**	**FOV**	**Slice Thick**	**Inter-space**	**NEX**	**TI**	**Pulse Sequence Options**
Sag PD FRFSE FS	3500	24	7	50	320	224	14/14	3	0	1		Sat S-I, F, FC, NPW
Sag T1 FSE	1050	24	4	41.67	288	192	14/14	3	0	2		Sat S-I, NPW
Ax PD FRFSE FS	3200	24	6	50	320	224	14/14	3.5	1	2		Sat S-I, F, FC, NPW
Cor PD-T2 FSE FS	3500	Min/ 80	16	50	320	224	14/14	3.5	.5	2		Sat S-I, F, FC, NPW

T1 FSE ETL 4 of lower.

TRF (Tailor Radio-Frequency) should be used with all FSE sequences to increase # of slices per TR.

Use NPW when possibility of anatomy wrapping (No Phase Wrap)

IDEAL can be used available (see grab bag in spine section)

Table 4-6   Site Protocol: Routine Knee

Sequence 1.5	TR	TE	ETL or FA	Band-width	F Matrix	Ph Matrix	FOV	Slice Thick	Inter-space	NEX	TI	Pulse Sequence Options

| Table 4-6 | Site Protocol: Routine Knee—*cont'd* |

Sequence 3T	TR	TE	ETL or FA	Band-width	F Matrix	Ph Matrix	FOV	Slice Thick	Inter-space	NEX	TI	Pulse Sequence Options

MRI OF THE LOWER LEG

Acquire three-plane pilot per site specifications.

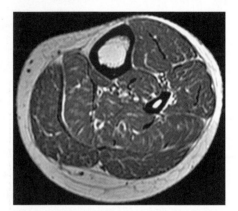

Figure 4-37 Axial image of the lower leg

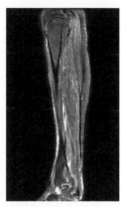

Figure 4-38 Sagittal image of the lower leg

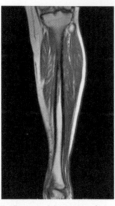

Figure 4-39 Coronal image of the lower leg

COIL: Vendor-specific multi-channel torso coil or cardiac coil
POSITION: Supine, feet first
LANDMARK: Midshaft of the tibia
IMMOBILIZATION: Surround the limb with sponges, place the ankle in a cushion to prevent rotation while scanning, and secure the extremity with Velcro straps.

> **TIP:** Use long-bone protocol. FOV is determined by the anatomy to be covered.
> If off-center FOV diminishes adequate fat saturation, STIR should be performed.

Acquisition of Coronal Image of the Lower Leg

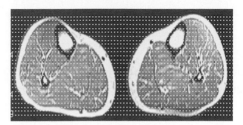

Figure 4-40 Axial image of the lower leg with coronal locations

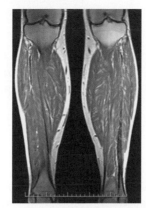

Figure 4-41 Coronal image of the lower leg

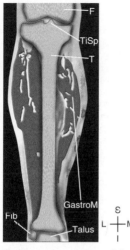

Figure 4-42 Coronal anatomy of the lower leg

KEY: **F**, femur; **Fib**, fibula; **GastroM**, gastrocnemius muscle; **T**, tibia; **TiSp**, spinal process of tibia.

SLICE ACQUISITION: Anterior to posterior

SLICE ALIGNMENT: Parallel to the shaft of the tibia

ANATOMIC COVERAGE: From femoral condyles to the calcaneus, including all musculature

TIP: Reference axial image to ensure that images are true coronals. This sequence is acquired bilaterally for comparison unless unilateral is requested by the physician. Place saturation pulse in saturation in the FOV to reduce vascular motion.

Acquisition of Axial Image of the Lower Leg

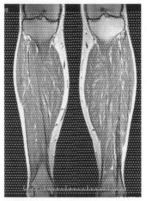

Figure 4-43 Coronal image of the lower leg with axial locs

SLICE ACQUISITION: Superior to inferior
SLICE ALIGNMENT: Perpendicular to the shaft of the tibia
ANATOMIC COVERAGE: From the femoral condoles through the calcaneus

TIP: This sequence can be prescribed unilaterally when requested by physician.

Figure 4-44 Axial image of the lower leg

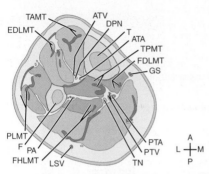

Figure 4-45 Axial anatomy of the lower leg

KEY: **ATA**, anterior tibial artery; **ATV**, anterior tibial vein; **DPN**, deep peroneal nerve; **EDLMT**, extensor digitorum longus muscle and tendon; **F**, fibula; **FDLMT**, flexor digitorum longus muscle and tendon; **FHLMT**, flexor hallucis longus muscle and tendon; **GS**, greatest saphenous; **LSV**, lesser saphenous vein; **PA**, peroneal artery; **PLMT**, peroneus longus muscle and tendon; **PTA**, posterior tibial artery; **PTV**, posterior tibial veins; **T**, tibia; **TAMT**, tibialis anterior muscle and tendon; **TN**, tibial nerve; **TPMT**, tibialis posterior muscle and tendon.

Acquisition of Sagittal Image of the Lower Leg

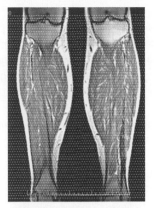

Figure 4-46 Coronal image of the lower leg with sagittal locations

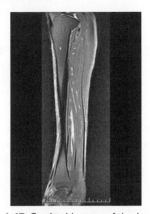

Figure 4-47 Sagittal image of the lower leg

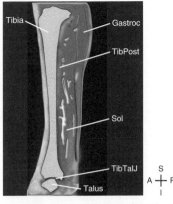

Figure 4-48 Sagittal anatomy of the lower leg

KEY: **Gastroc**, gastrocnemius; **Sol**, soleus muscle; **TibPost**, tibialis posterior muscle; **TipTalJ**, tibial talar joint.

SLICE ACQUISITION: Lateral to medial
SLICE ALIGNMENT: Parallel to the shaft of the tibia
ANATOMIC COVERAGE: From the femoral condyles to the calcaneus

TIP: This sequence is prescribed unilaterally unless bilateral is requested by the physician.
Always reference axial image to ensure proper alignment. Saturation pulse in the FOV to reduce vascular motion (see Table 4-3, long bone protocol).

MRI OF THE ANKLE

Acquire three-plane pilot per site specifications.

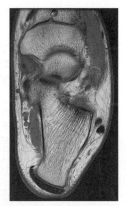

Figure 4-49 Axial image of the ankle

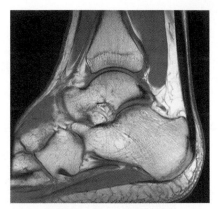

Figure 4-50 Sagittal image of the ankle

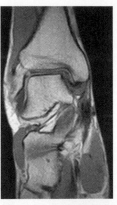

Figure 4-51 Coronal image of the ankle

COIL: Multi-channel vendor-specific extremity coil
POSITION: Supine, feet first
LANDMARK: At level of lateral malleolus
IMMOBILIZATION: Secure the foot on all sides with cushions, and place cushions under
the lower leg to support the knee and calf.

Acquisition of Axial Images of the Ankle

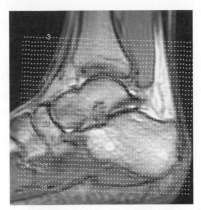

Figure 4-52 Sagittal image of the ankle with axial locations

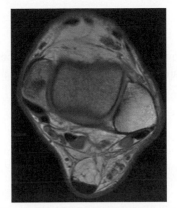

Figure 4-53 Axial image of the ankle

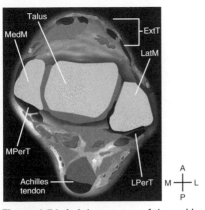

Figure 4-54 Axial anatomy of the ankle

SLICE ACQUISITION: Superior to inferior
SLICE ALIGNMENT: Parallel to the tibiotalar joint (ankle mortise)
ANATOMIC COVERAGE: From the distal tibia through the calcaneus

KEY: **ExtT**, extensor tendons; **LatM**, lateral malleolus; **LPerT**, lateral peroneal tendon; **MedM**, medial malleolus; **MPerT**, medial peroneal tendon.

TIP: Reference the coronal image to ensure that slices are parallel to the ankle mortise.
  Saturation in the FOV to reduce vascular motion.

Acquisition of Sagittal Images of the Ankle

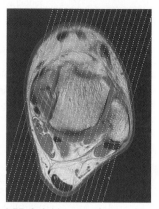

Figure 4-55 Axial image of the ankle with sagittal locations

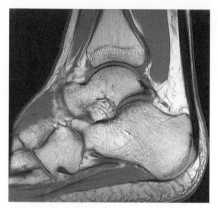

Figure 4-56 Sagittal image of the ankle

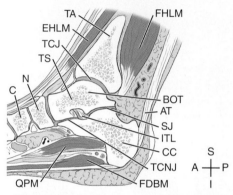

Figure 4-57 Sagittal anatomy of the ankle

KEY: AT, Achilles tendon; **BOT**, body of talus; **C**, cuneiform; **CC**, calcaneous; **EHLM**, extensor hallucis longus muscle; **FDBM**, flexor digitorum brevis muscle; **FHLM**, flexor hallucis longus muscle; **ITL**, interosseous talocalcaneal ligament; **N**, navicular; **QPM**, quadratus plantae muscle; **SJ**, subtalar joint; **TA**, tibia; **TCJ**, talocrural joint; **TCNJ**, talocalcaneonavicular joint; **TS**, talus.

SLICE ACQUISITION: Lateral to medial
SLICE ALIGNMENT: Parallel to the talofibular joint
ANATOMIC COVERAGE: From the lateral malleolus of the fibula to the medial malleolus of the tibia, from the distal tibia through the calcaneus and surrounding musculature

TIP: Reference the sagittal pilot to ensure coverage through the calcaneal tuberosity for Achilles tendon tear.
Saturation (superior) in the FOV to reduce vascular motion.

Acquisition of Coronal Images of the Ankle

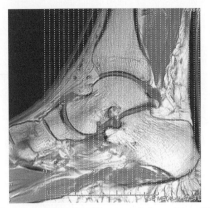

Figure 4-58 Sagittal image of the ankle with coronal locations

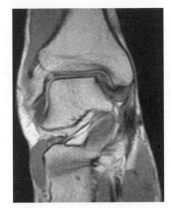

Figure 4-59 Coronal image of the ankle

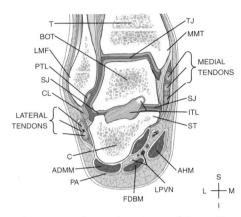

Figure 4-60 Coronal anatomy of the ankle

SLICE ACQUISITION: Anterior to posterior

SLICE ALIGNMENT: Perpendicular to the tibiotalar joint (ankle mortise)

ANATOMIC COVERAGE: From proximal metatarsals to calcaneal tuberosity, including the Achilles tendon, from the distal tibia through the calcaneal tuberosity

TIP: Saturation (superior) in the FOV to reduce vascular motion

KEY: **ADMM**, abductor digiti minimi muscle; **AHM**, abductor hallucis muscle; **BOT**, body of talus; **C**, calcaneus; **CL**, calcaneofibular ligament; **FDBM**, flexor digitorum brevis muscle; **IFR**, inferior fibular retinaculum; **ITL**, interosseous talocalcaneal joint; **LMF**, lateral malleolus of fibula; **LPVN**, lateral plantar vessels and nerve; **MMT**, medial malleolus of tibia; **PA**, plantar aponeurosis; **PTL**, posterior talofibular ligament; **SJ**, subtalar joint (talocalcaneal joint); **ST**, sustentaculum tail; **T**, tibia.

| Table 4-7 | Routine Ankle |

Sequence 1.5	TR	TE	ETL or FA	Band-width	F Matrix	Ph Matrix	FOV	Slice Thick	Inter-space	NEX	TI	Pulse Sequence Options
Sag IR	3000	50	5	41.67	256	192	14-16	3.0	.5	2	150	Sat S-I, FC, seq, NPW
Sag T1 FSE	550	Min	4	41.67	448	224	14-16	3.0	.5	2		Sat S-I, NPW
AX PD FSE FS	3500	25	9	41.67	256	224	14-16	4.0	1.0	3		Sat S-I, F, Zip 512
AX T1 FSE	600	Min	3	31.25	256	224	14-16	4.0	1.0	2		Sat S-I
Cor IT FSE	3500	65	11	41.67	256	192	14-16	3.5	0	2	150	Sat S-I, FC, seq

Table 4-7 Routine Ankle—*cont'd*

Sequence 3T	TR	TE	ETL or FA	Band-width	F Matrix	Ph Matrix	FOV	Slice Thick	Inter-space	NEX	TI	Pulse Sequence Options
Sag IR FSE	4000	50	23	50	256	192	12-14	3.0	.5	2	190	Sat S-I, FC, seq, NPW
SAG T1 FSE	1100	Min	4	83.33	448	224	12-14	3.0	.5	2		Sat S-I, NPW
AX PD FSE FS	3000	25	11	50	384	224	12/12	3.0	.5	3		Sat S-I, F, FC
AX T1 FSE	1100	Min	4	83.33	448	224	12/12	3.0	.5	2		Sat S-I
Cor IR FSE	4000	50	23	50	256	192	12/12	3.0	.5	2	190	Sat S-I, FC, seq

T1 FSE ETL 4 of lower.
TRF (Tailor Radio-Frequency) should be used with all FSE sequences to increase # of slices per TR.
Use NPW when possibility of anatomy wrapping (No Phase Wrap)
IDEAL can be used available (see grab bag in spine section)

Table 4-8 Site Protocol: Routine Ankle

Sequence 1.5	TR	TE	ETL or FA	Band-width	F Matrix	Ph Matrix	FOV	Slice Thick	Inter-space	NEX	TI	Pulse Sequence Options

Sequence 3T	TR	TE	ETL or FA	Band-width	F Matrix	Ph Matrix	FOV	Slice Thick	Inter-space	NEX	TI	Pulse Sequence Options

Table 4-8 Site Protocol: Routine Ankle—*cont'd*

MRI OF THE FOOT AND DIGITS

Acquire three-plane pilots per site specifications.
For individual digits, follow the same protocol as for the foot, using a reduced FOV.

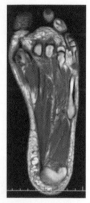

Figure 4-61 Axial image of the foot

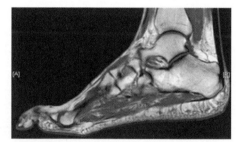

Figure 4-62 Sagittal image of the foot

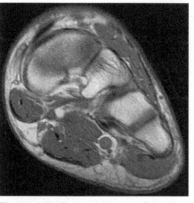

Figure 4-63 Coronal image of the foot

COIL: Multi-channel vendor-specific foot and ankle coil. Knee coil with chimney may be used.

POSITION: Supine, feet first

LANDMARK: Midmetatarsals

IMMOBILIZATION: Secure the foot on all sides with cushions, place an angle wedge against the toes to prevent motion during the scan, and place cushions under the lower leg to support the knee and calf.

Acquisition of Axial (Long-Axis) Images of the Foot

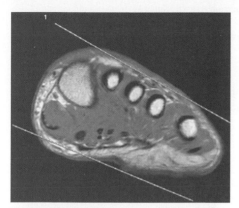

Figure 4-64 Sagittal image of the foot with axial locations

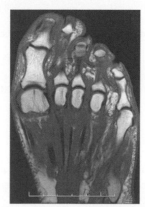

Figure 4-65 Axial image of the foot

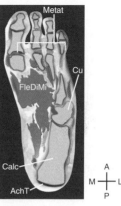

Figure 4-66 Axial anatomy of the foot

KEY: **AchT**, Achilles tendon; **Calc**, calcaneus; **Cu**, cuboid; **FleDiMi**, flexor digital minimus; **Metat**, metatarsals.

SLICE ACQUISITION: Superior to inferior

SLICE ALIGNMENT: Parallel to the metatarsals

ANATOMIC COVERAGE: From anterior through the plantar fascia, from the most distal phalanx through the calcaneus

TIP: The long axis is usually considered the axial of the foot. Reference the three-plane pilot to ensure adequate anatomic coverage.

Acquisition of Coronal (Short-Axis) Images of the Foot

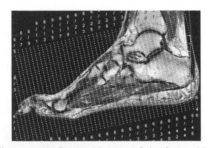

Figure 4-67 Sagittal image of the foot with coronal locations

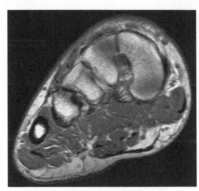

Figure 4-68 Coronal image of the foot

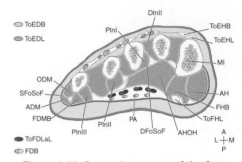

Figure 4-69 Coronal anatomy of the foot

SLICE ACQUISITION: Distal to proximal

SLICE ALIGNMENT: Perpendicular to the metatarsals

ANATOMIC COVERAGE: From the most distal phalanx though the calcaneus, including the plantar fascia

TIP: Short axis is usually considered coronal of the foot. Reference the three-plane pilot to ensure adequate anatomic coverage.

Superior saturation pulse in the FOV to reduce vascular motion.

KEY: AH, abductor hallucis; **ADM,** abductor digit minimi; **AHOH,** abductor hallucis, oblique head; **FHB,** flexor hallucis brevis; **FDMB,** flexor digit minimi brevis; **FDB,** flexor digitorum brevis; **MI,** metatarsal I; **ODM,** opponens digit minimi; **PA,** plantar aponeurosis; **PInI,** plantar interosseus I; **PInII,** plantar interosseus II; **PInIII,** plantar interosseus III; **SFoSoF,** superior fascia of sole of foot; **ToEDB,** tendons of extensor digitorum brevis; **ToEDL,** tendons of extensor digitorum longus; **ToFDLaL,** tendons of flexor digitorum longus and lumbricals; **ToEHL,** tendons of extensor hallucis longus; **ToEHB,** tendon of extensor hallucis brevis; **ToFHL,** tendon of flexor hallucis longus.

Acquisition of Sagittal Images of the Foot

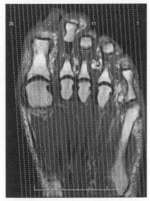

Figure 4-70 Axial image of the foot with sagittal locations

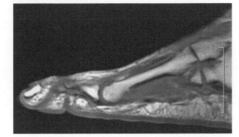

Figure 4-71 Sagittal image of the foot

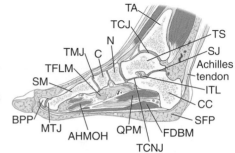

Figure 4-72 Sagittal anatomy of the foot

SLICE ACQUISITION: Lateral to medial

SLICE ALIGNMENT: Parallel to the metatarsals

ANATOMIC COVERAGE: From fifth metatarsal to first metatarsal, including the distal phalanx to the calcaneus

TIP: Saturation (superior) in the FOV to reduce vascular motion.

KEY: **AHMOH**, adductor hallucis muscle, oblique head; **BPP**, base of proximal phalanx; **C**, cuneiform; **CC**, calcaneous; **FDBM**, flexor digitorum brevis muscle; **ITL**, interosseous talocalcaneal ligament; **MTJ**, metatarsophalangeal joint; **N**, navicular; **QPM**, quadratus plantae muscle; **SFP**, subcalcaneal fat pad; **SJ**, subtalar joint; **SM**, second metatarsal; **TA**, tibia; **TCJ**, talocrural joint; **TCNJ**, talocalcaneonavicular joint; **TFLM**, tendon of fibularis longus muscle; **TMJ**, tarsometatarsal joint; **TS**, talus.

Table 4-9 Routine Foot

Sequence 1.5	TR	TE	ETL or FA	Band-width	F Matrix	Ph Matrix	FOV	Slice Thick	Inter-space	NEX	TI	Pulse Sequence Options
SAG FSE IR	3000	50	11	41.67	256	192	12-14	3.0	.5	3	150	Sat S-I, FC, seq, NPW
SAG T1 FSE	450	Min	4	31.25	320	224	12-14	3.0	.5	2		Sat S-I, NPW
Cor PD FRFSE FS	3500	25	7	41.67	320	224	12-14	3.0	.5	2		Sat S-I, F, FC
COR T1 FSE	700	Min	4	31.25	320	224	12-14	3.0	.5	2		Sat S-I,
AX IR FSE	4000	50	23	41.67	256	192	12-14	3.0	0	4	150	Sat S-I, FC, seq
AX T1 FSE	800	Min	4	50	448	224	12-14	3.0	0	1		Sat S-I, TRF

Table 4-9				Routine Foot—*cont'd*								
Sequence 3T	TR	TE	ETL or FA	Band-width	F Matrix	Ph Matrix	FOV	Slice Thick	Inter-space	NEX	TI	Pulse Sequence Options
SAG FSE IR	4500	68	17	50	384	192	12-14	3.0	0	2	190-200	Sat S-I, FC, Seq, NPW
SAG T1 FSE	875	Min	4	50	512	224	12-14	3.0	0	2		Sat S-I, TRF, NPW
Cor PD FRFSE FS	3200	32	7	62.50	384	224	10-12	5.0	.5	2		Sat S-I, F, FC
COR T1 FSE	925	Min	4	50	448	224	10-12	5.0	.5	2		Sat S-I
AX IR FSE	4000	50	23	83.33	448	224	12-14	3.0	0	3	190-200	Sat S-I, FC, seq
AX T1 FSE	800	Min	4	50	448	224	12-14	3.0	0	1		Sat S-I

T1 FSE ETL 4 of lower.

For entire foot increase the FOV.

TRF (Tailor Radio-Frequency) should be used with all FSE sequences to increase # of slices per TR.

Use NPW when possibility of anatomy wrapping (No Phase Wrap)

IDEAL can be used available (see grab bag in spine section)

Table 4-10 Site Protocol: Routine Foot

Sequence 1.5	TR	TE	ETL or FA	Band-width	F Matrix	Ph Matrix	FOV	Slice Thick	Inter-space	NEX	TI	Pulse Sequence Options

Sequence 3T	TR	TE	ETL or FA	Band-width	F Matrix	Ph Matrix	FOV	Slice Thick	Inter-space	NEX	TI	Pulse Sequence Options

Table 4-10 Site Protocol: Routine Foot—*cont'd*

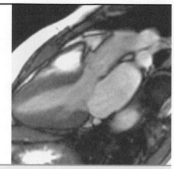

CHAPTER 5

MRI of the Thorax

CHAPTER OUTLINE

MRI OF THE BREAST

Scan Considerations

MRI has a role in the detection and management of *some* breast cancers. Routine mammography can miss two of three breast cancers. Because of increased vascularity, breast malignancies typically enhance brighter and more intensely than benign tissues after intravenous injection of contrast. It is imperative to scan both breasts simultaneously in about 90 seconds per phase to evaluate for breast cancer. All vendors offer high-definition bilateral volume breast imaging, which makes this possible.

The GE VIBRANT (Volume Imaging for BReast AssessmeNT), or vendor equivalent, allows you to perform bilateral breast examinations in both the sagittal and axial planes. VIBRANT is a high-resolution fast spoiled gradient echo (T1) with ASSET (parallel imaging) and "Special," a fat-saturation technique that uses an inversion recovery pulse to eliminate fat. The scan time with VIBRANT is equal to the scan time of a single-breast scan in the past. It obtains high temporal resolution without sacrificing spatial resolution. VIBRANT eliminates fat to enhance and better identify lesions.

Patient Preparation and Positioning

Patients are screened with both MRI screening and a breast screening form. The patient's history and pertinent mammogram and ultrasound imaging information are important for radiologist interpretation.

Breast MR is menstrual cycle and hormone dependent. Breast MR is best performed in midcycle (week 2, day 7-14). Imaging the patient at this optimal time in her cycle does not completely exclude enhancement of benign breast parenchyma. Benign background hormonal enhancement is one of the greatest challenges facing interpretation of breast MR in premenopausal women.

The patient is prepared with a 22-G or less intravenous line in the antecubital vein. A dose of 0.1 mmol per kilogram of body weight of gadolinium contrast is suggested (see Contrast section). A power injector should be prepared with contrast and 20 mL of saline. The suggested flow rate is 2 mL/second for contrast and 2 mL/second for saline. An injector delay is determined at the time of scanning to allow for a mask and additional postcontrast phases. *Timing is essential.*

Before positioning the patient, breast markers should be placed on the patient's nipples and any scars or biopsy sites. The technologist should explain the examination to the patient and emphasize the importance of holding still and not changing position, particularly between pre- and postcontrast scans. The patient is positioned prone in a high-

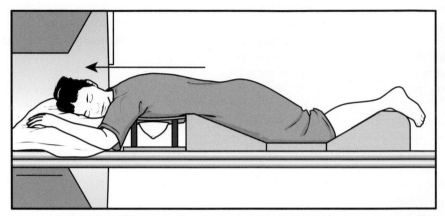

Figure 5-1 Correct positioning in dedicated bilateral breast coil

definition (HD) breast coil. High-definition breast array coils are available from all vendors and have biopsy capabilities. The breasts should be hanging freely in the coil and not touching the sides. Place gauze between the patient and the coil when necessary to avoid any possibility of bright signal from coil burnout. The patient should be made as comfortable as possible, making sure to support the feet as well as the head and arms. Communicating with the patient during the examination is imperative. The patient's intravenous line should be hooked up to the power injector before the examination begins.

A typical bilateral breast examination is composed of a calibration scan, which must extend past anatomy by 50% superiorly and inferiorly. FOV is patient-dependent Bilateral shim volumes should be applied, covering as much of the breasts as possible and taking care not to include the heart or lungs. A three-dimensional VIBRANT (T1 FSPGR) axial non–fat-saturated scan is acquired to evaluate the fatty structures of the breast. The axial plane is preferred for bilateral evaluation by the radiologist. Multiphase pre- and post-VIBRANT scans with "special" (spatial fat saturation) are performed, which include a mask and five or six post-contrast phases.

The phase timing is determined by the VIBRANT non–fat-saturated scan. Autosubtraction is imperative to remove pre-contrast tissue. A sagittal VIBRANT post-contrast delayed scan should be performed. Sagittal T2 fat-saturation scans can be performed bilaterally as well as a bilateral axial T2 fat-saturation or STIR. Fat and water separation imaging, IDEAL, can be used to replace all fat-saturated imaging. The total scan time is around 30 to 45 minutes.

The technologist and nurse must be "in synch." The programmable "inject delay time" should be doubled-checked to ensure that it is correct. The technologist should inform the patient of the injection before it is administered, reinforcing the importance of holding still. *Timing is everything* in breast imaging.

Evaluation of contrast image enhancement is important to determine lesion kinetics. This can help to determine malignant from nonmalignant lesions. Image timing is extremely important because malignant lesions can enhance and wash out their contrast in about 90 seconds. The "time-intensity curve" of dynamic phases can help determine malignant from benign. Computer-assisted diagnosis (CAD) for MR is available from several vendors. These systems provide time-intensity curves, multiplanar reformatting, and subtraction imaging options;

angiogenesis maps; maximum intensity projections (MIP); volume summaries; and vascular maximum intensity projection images.

To evaluate a region of interest, a cursor is placed over the focally enhanced area, and a kinetic curve is produced and evaluated. In the early post-contrast phase (60 to 90 seconds after injection), the washout rate, or enhancement velocity, is quantified. Radiologists routinely analyze both the morphologic features of the lesion and the kinetic curves. Morphologic features are reliable tools in diagnosis and treatment planning.

Sequence Significance

Nonenhanced, nonfat saturation VIBRANT (T1-SPGR) images identify high signal hemorrhagic or proteinaceous cysts and high signal proteinaceous material within dilated ducts.

VIBRANT pre-contrast images are subtracted from the post-contrast images so only areas of enhancement are prominent.

Because both fat and water can appear bright on T2, fat-saturated sequences are performed. T2 fat saturation and/or STIR are used to determine high-signal masses such as cysts, lymph nodes, or fibroadenomas. Carcinomas are usually isointense or hypointense in this sequence.

Bilateral Breast Imaging

Acquire three-plane pilot per site specifications.

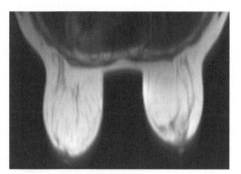

Figure 5-2 Axial breast

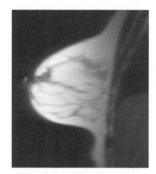

Figure 5-3 Sagittal breast

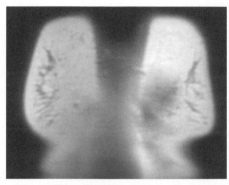

Figure 5-4 Coronal breast

COIL: Multi-channel vendor-specific breast coil
POSITION: Prone, feet first with the breasts suspended in the coil
Place the cushion under the ankles, with the arms extended comfortably toward the head.
LANDMARK: Midcoil
IMMOBILIZATION: Shield the patient from touching the sides of the magnet by using
   sponges or sheet.

TIP: Place MR markers on the patient's nipples and surgical scar sites before positioning.

Acquisition of Axial images of the Breasts

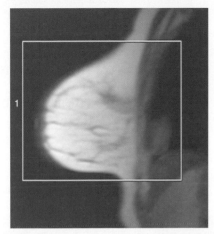

Figure 5-5 Sagittal image of the breast with axial locations

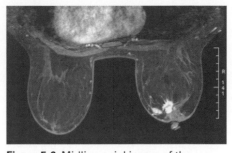

Figure 5-6 Midline axial image of the breasts

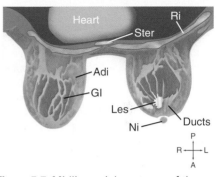

Figure 5-7 Midline axial anatomy of the breasts

KEY: Adi, adipose; **Gl**, glandular lobule; **Les**, lesion; **Ni**, nipple; **Ri**, rib; **Ster**, sternum.

SLICE ACQUISITION: Plot superior to inferior
SLICE ALIGNMENT: Perpendicular to the sternum
ANATOMIC COVERAGE: Chest wall through the nipple, including the axillary margins

TIP: Breasts are often asymmetric. Cross-reference bilateral sagittal pilots to ensure complete coverage of both breasts. An additional post-contrast VIBRANT without using SPF (swap phase and frequency) will best visualize the axilla.

Acquisition of Sagittal Images of the Breasts

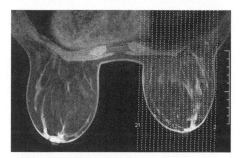

Figure 5-8 Axial image of the breast with sagittal locations

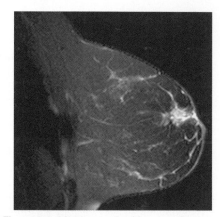

Figure 5-9 Midline sagittal image of a single breast

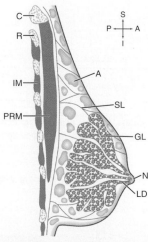

Figure 5-10 Midline sagittal anatomy of the breast

KEY: A, adipose; **C**, clavicle; **GL**, glandular lobule; **IM**, intercostal muscle; **LD**, lactiferous duct; **N**, nipple; **PRM**, pectoralis major muscle; **R**, rip; **SL**, suspensory ligament.

SLICE ACQUISITION: For bilateral three-dimensional acquisitions, scan left to right through both breasts.

SLICE ALIGNMENT: Straight, no angle

ANATOMIC COVERAGE: Midthoracic cavity to the nipples, including the axillary margins

TIP: Breasts are often asymmetric. Cross-reference axial pilots to ensure complete coverage of both breasts.

Table 5-1 MRI of the Breast

Sequence 1.5	TR	TE	ETL or FA	Band-width	F Matrix	Ph Matrix	FOV	Slice Thick	Inter-space	NEX	TI	Pulse Sequence Options
Axial Vibrant C			10 FA	41.67	320	320	32-36	1.8	0	1	96 loc/slab	3-D Vibrant, Zip 2, Sat A, SPF
Post GAD												
Axial Vibrant C-/+			10 FA	62.50	384	320	32-36	1.8	0	1	96 loc/slab	3-D Vibrant, Zip 2, Multi-phase, Special, SPF
Sagittal Vibrant			10 FA	41.67	256	224	18-20	2.4	0	1	110 loc/slab	3-D fast Vibrant, Zip 2, Special, NPW
Sag T2 FSE FS	4000	102	17 ETL	41.67	256	224	20/20	4	1	2		Sat F, FC NPW
Ax FSE IR	6000	32	9 ETL	31.25	320	192	32-36	5	1	1	150	Asset, FC, seq
Delayed Ax Vibrant			10 FA	41.67	320	370	32-36	1.8	0	1	96 loc/slab	3-D Vibrant, Zip 2, Special
OPT Brease	2000	155					36/36	20		32		MRS, Sat R-L-A-P

(Continued)

| Table 5-1 | MRI of the Breast—cont'd |

Sequence 3T	TR	TE	ETL or FA	Band-width	F Matrix	Ph Matrix	FOV	Slice Thick	Inter-space	NEX	TI	Pulse Sequence Options
Axial Vibrant C			10 FA	83.33	388	388	32-36	1.8	0	1	100 loc/ slab	3-D Vibrant, Zip 2, Sat A, SPF
Post GAD												
Axial Vibrant C-/+			10 FA	83.33	388	388	32-36	1.8	0	1	100 loc/ slab	3-D Vibrant, Zip 2, Multi-phase, Special, SPF
Sag Vibrant			10 FA	83.33	256	256	18/20	2.0	0	1	160 loc/ slab	3-D Vibrant, Zip 2, Special, NPW
Sag T2 FSE FS	4700	120	17 ETL	50	256	224	20/20	4	1	2		Sat F, FC NPW, Zip 512
Ax FSE IR	6000	32	9 ETL	62.50	384	224	32/36	5	1	1	175	Asset, FC, TRF, Seq
Delayed Ax Vibrant			10 FA	83.33	388	388	32-36	1.8	0	1	100 loc/ slab	3D Vibrant, Zip 2, Sat A
OPT Brease	2000	155					36/36	20		32		MRS, Sat R-L-A-P

TR and TE are machine dependent. Loc/slab and FOV is patient dependent.
Delayed axial vibrant is performed without SPF to move flow artifact and best visualize the axilla.
TRF (Tailor Radio-Frequency) should be used with all FSE sequence to increase # of slices per TR.
Can use IDEAL when availabel (see grab bag). Brease is GE spectroscopy of the breast.

Table 5-2 Site Protocol: MRI of the Breast

Sequence 1.5	TR	TE	ETL or FA	Band-width	F Matrix	Ph Matrix	FOV	Slice Thick	Inter-space	NEX	TI	Pulse Sequence Options
Post GAD												

Sequence 3T	TR	TE	ETL or FA	Band-width	F Matrix	Ph Matrix	FOV	Slice Thick	Inter-space	NEX	TI	Pulse Sequence Options
Post GAD												

CARDIAC MRI

Cardiac Nomenclature

In 2002 the Cardiac Imaging Committee of the Council on Clinical Cardiology of the American Heart Association issued a statement for health care professionals. In an effort to standardize the nomenclature for cardiac imaging, they recommended "all imaging modalities should define, orient and display the heart using the long axis of the left ventricle and selected planes oriented at 90-degrees angles relative to the long axis" (Manuel D, et al: Standardized myocardial segmentation and nomenclature for tomographic imaging of the heart, *Circulation 105:* 539, 2002).

The nomenclature of short, vertical long, and horizontal long axis is suggested for cardiac planes used in cardiac MR. For the purpose of industry-wide consistency, this nomenclature will be adhered to in this text. See Figure 5-11 below.

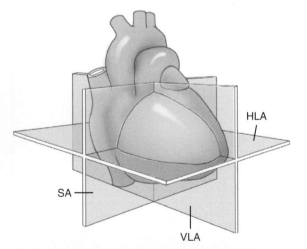

KEY: **HLA**, horizontal line axis; **SA**, short axis; **VLA**, vertical line axis.

KEY: **A**, aorta; **ASV**, aortic semilunar valve; **BA**, bicuspid (mitral) (left atrioventricular) valve; **BT**, brachiocephalic trunk; **En**, endocardium; **Ep**, epicardium; **IS**, interventricular septum; **IVC**, inferior vena cava; **LA**, left atrium; **LCCA**, left common carotid artery; **LSA**, left subclavian artery; **LV**, left ventricle; **M**, myocardium; **PA**, pulmonary artery; **PSV**, pulmonary semilunar valve; **PV**, pulmonary veins; **RA**, right atrium; **RV**, right ventricle; **SVC**, superior vena cava; **TV**, tricuspid (right atrioventricular) valve.

Figure 5-11 Planes of the heart

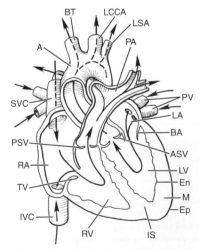

Figure 5-12 Chambers of the heart

Scan Considerations

- A detailed cardiac history including any and all surgical interventions must be established before scanning.
- The importance of the patient holding their breath, and the patient's capability to do so, must be assessed and discussed before scanning the patient.
- All breath-hold sequences are acquired during a single-breath-hold on expiration, including the calibration scan.
- A considerable amount of cardiac imaging is done using FIESTA (fast imaging employing steady-state acquisition), a gated cine sequence.
- FIESTA is a gated bright blood sequence used for all planes, i.e., short-axis; long-axis; 2-, 3-, and 4-chamber studies.
- Double IR is a TI blood-suppressed image (black blood).
- Triple IR is a TI blood-suppressed, fat saturated image (black blood with fat saturation).
- PC (phased contrast) imaging is used to identify and measure flow within a vessel. It uses velocity encoding (VENC) to visualize the flow within a vessel. The VENC of the aorta is approximately 200-250 cm/sec and the VENC of the pulmonary artery is approximately 150-200 cm/sec.
- Delayed enhancement is an IR prep sequence that visualizes defects in the myocardium. When scanning, the TI must be adjusted to maximize nullification of the myocardium.
- Scan times are heart rate and patient dependent.
- FOV is dependent on the patient's size.
- MRA of the aorta can be performed as a gated or non-gated sequence.
- Zoom gradients should always be used when available. When used, it decreases the TE, which is necessary in all steady-state imaging because minimum TR/TE is desirable.
- A small volume shim is placed directly over the heart and should be checked in all 3 planes before scanning.

Gating

Most cardiac sequences require synchronization with the cardiac cycle—thus the need for cardiac gating. Because of the magnetohydrodymanic effect, elevated T waves can cause false triggering if standard amplitude-based electrocardiographic leads are used. Magnetohydrodymanic effect is a type of oscillation of plasma particles consisting of transverse waves propagating along the magnetic field lines in plasma. T-wave swelling can be so large that the amplitude of the T wave is greater than that of the R wave, resulting in incorrect triggering of the MR sequence. For this reason, VCG is recommended. With VCG gating, lead pairs measure voltages that are orthogonal to one another. All MR vendors provide general guidelines for correct lead placement, however, the general placement for accurate VCG gating is shown below.

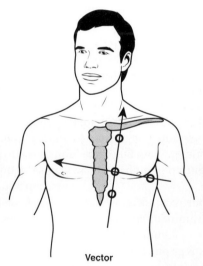

Vector

Figure 5-13 VCG lead placement

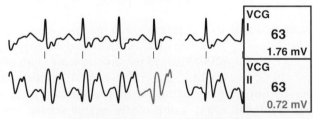

Figure 5-14 Example of VCG display

Cardiac Imaging

Acquire a three-plane pilot per site specifications.

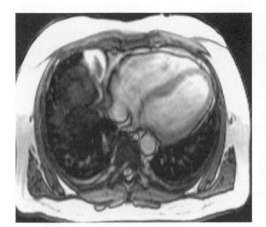

Figure 5-15 Axial image of the heart

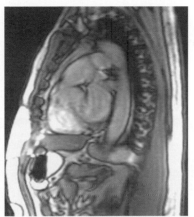

Figure 5-16 Sagittal image of the heart

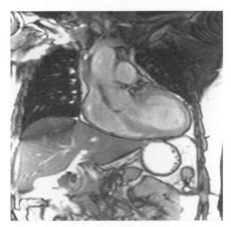

Figure 5-17 Coronal image of the heart

COIL: Vendor-specific multi-channel cardiac coil
POSITION: Supine, feet first with arms resting at sides
LANDMARK: Midcoil, xiphoid
IMMOBILIZATION: Support the arms and knees with cushions. Prevent the body from touching the sides of the magnet by using sponges or sheets.

TIP: Use zoom gradient when available. Make sure the volume shim is placed directly over the heart.

Acquisition of Long-Axis Localizer

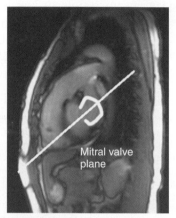

Figure 5-18 Sagittal image with location from the apex to the mitral valve

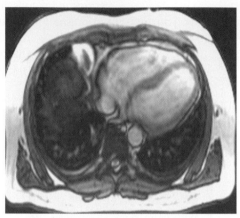

Figure 5-19 Vertical long-axis image

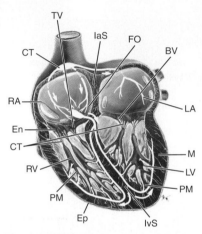

Figure 5-20 Vertical long-axis anatomy

SLICE ACQUISITION: Inferior to superior

SLICE ALIGNMENT: Follow the long axis of the heart bisecting the left ventricular apex and mitral valve plane.

ANATOMIC COVERAGE: Entire heart, thoracic cavity, ribs to spine

KEY: **BV**, bicuspid value; **CT**, chordae tendinae; **En**, endocardium, **Ep**, epicardium; **FO**, fossa ovalis; **IaS**, interatrial septum; **IvS**, interventricular septum; **LA**, left atrium; **LV**, left ventricle; **M**, myocardium; **PM**, papillary muscle; **RA**, right atrium; **RV**, right ventricle; **TV**, tricuspid value.

Acquisition of Short-Axis Images of the Heart

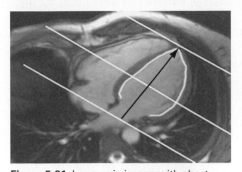

Figure 5-21 Long-axis image with short axis locs

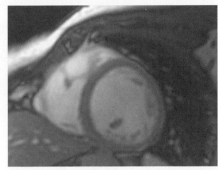

Figure 5-22 Short axis image of the heart

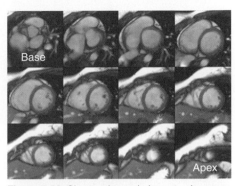

Figure 5-23 Short-axis stack, base to the apex of the heart

SLICE ACQUISITION: Posterior to anterior
SLICE ALIGNMENT: Perpendicular to the septum and left ventricular wall
ANATOMIC COVERAGE: From base to apex

TIP: Use zoom gradient when available. Make sure the volume shim is placed directly over the heart.

Each slice is acquired during a single breath hold. Instruct the patient to stop breathing at the end of expiration.

Long-Axis Imaging of the Heart: Two-, Three-, and Four-Chamber Studies
Acquisition of Two-Chamber Study

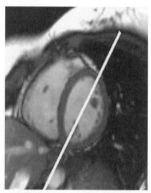

Figure 5-24 Short-axis image at midventricle with location for two-chamber study

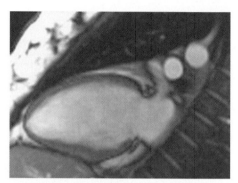

Figure 5-25 Two-chamber image

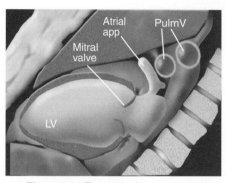

Figure 5-26 Two-chamber anatomy

SLICE ACQUISITION: Single cine image to demonstrate the motion of the anterior and inferior walls

SLICE ALIGNMENT: Parallel to the septum bisecting the anterior and inferior walls of the left ventricle

ANATOMY DEMONSTRATED: Left ventricle, mitral valve, and left atrial appendage

KEY: **Atrial app**, atrial appendage; **LV**, left ventricle; **PulmV**, pulmonary veins.

TIP: Use zoom gradient when available. Make sure the volume shim is placed directly over the heart. Each slice is acquired during a single breath hold. Instruct the patient to stop breathing at the end of expiration.

Acquisition of Three-Chamber Study: Left Ventricular Outflow Tract

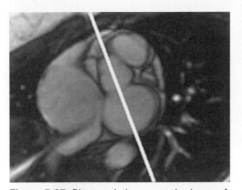

Figure 5-27 Short-axis image at the base of the heart bisecting the aortic outflow tract

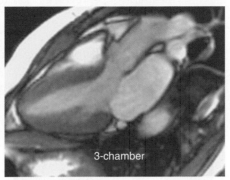

Figure 5-28 Left ventricular outflow tract

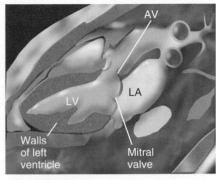

Figure 5-29 Anatomy of left ventricular outflow tract

SLICE ACQUISITION: Single cine image demonstrating left ventricular outflow tract

SLICE ALIGNMENT: Parallel to the aortic outflow tract

ANATOMY DEMONSTRATED: Walls of the left ventricle, mitral and aortic valves, and left atrium

KEY: **AV**, aortic valve; **LA**, left atrium; **LV**, left ventricle.

TIP: Use zoom gradient when available. Make sure the volume shim is placed directly over the heart. Each slice is acquired during a single breath hold. Instruct the patient to stop breathing at the end of expiration.

Acquisition of Four-Chamber Study

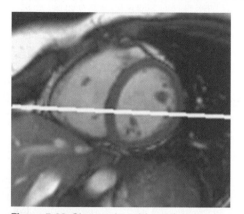

Figure 5-30 Short-axis, midventricle image bisecting the septum and right ventricle

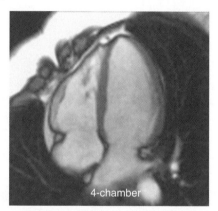

4-chamber

Figure 5-31 Four-chamber image

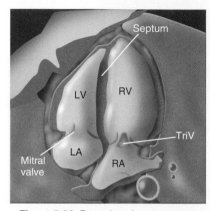

Figure 5-32 Four-chamber anatomy

KEY: LA, left atrium; **LV**, left ventricle; **RA**, right atrium; **RV**, right ventricle; **TriV**, tricuspid valve.

SLICE ACQUISITION: Single cine image

SLICE ALIGNMENT: Perpendicular to the septum at the highest curvature of the right ventricle

ANATOMY DEMONSTRATED: Right atrium, right ventricle, left atrium, left ventricle, mitral and tricuspid valves, septum

TIP: Use zoom gradient when available. Make sure the volume shim is placed directly over the heart.

Each slice is acquired during a single breath hold. Instruct the patient to stop breathing at the end of expiration.

MRA OF THE GREAT VESSELS OF THE THORAX

Myelography can be acquired in addition to MRI of the spine in the cervical, thoracic or lumber regions.

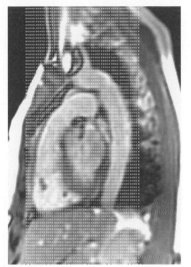

Figure 5-33 Sagittal chest with coronal loc for MRA of the thorax

COIL: Multi-channel Cardiac coil
POSITION: Supine, head first, cushion under kness
LANDMARK: Mid sternum

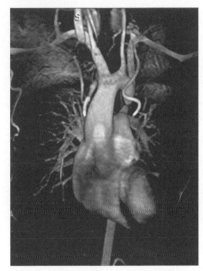

Figure 5-34 MRA of the thorax

KEY: AA, aortic arch; **BoRPA**, branch of right pulmonary artery; **BT**, brachiocephalic trunk; **DA**, descending aorta; **IG**, interventricular groove; **IVC**, inferior vena cava; **LA**, ligamentum arteriosum; **LBV**, left brachiocephalic vein; **LCCA**, left common carotid artery; **LIPV**, left inferior pulmonary vein; **LPA**, left pulmonary artery; **LSA**, left

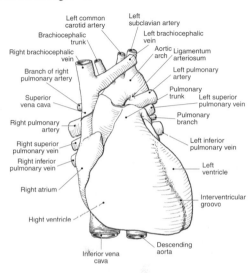

Figure 5-35 Vascular anatomy of the thorax

subclavian artery; **LSPV**, left superior pulmonary vein; **LV**, left ventricle; **PB**, pulmonary branch; **Pt**, pulmonary trunk; **RA**, right atrium; **RBV**, right brachiocephalic vein; **RIPV**, right inferior pulmonary vein; **RPA**, right pulmonary artery; **RSPV**, right superior pulmonary vein; **RV**, right ventricle; **SVC**, superior vena cava.

Table 5-3 Cardiac MRI

Sequence 1.5	TR	TE	ETL or FA	Band-width	F Matrix	Ph Matrix	FOV	Slice Thick	Inter-space	NEX	TI	Pulse Sequence Options
3-plane nongated fiesta loc	Min		60	125	192	160	40/40	8	0	1		2D Fiesta, Fast, Seq
Fiesta	Min	Min full	45 FA	125	192	160	36/36	8	0	1		Fiesta, Fast, Seq, Cine, ECG gated
Double IR FSE		42	32	62	256	256	30-40/.75	5-8		1	BSP Auto	Gating, Seq, BSP, Zip 512, #RR 2, Trigger Delay Min

| **Table 5-3** | Cardiac MRI—cont'd |

Sequence 1.5	TR	TE	ETL or FA	Band-width	F Matrix	Ph Matrix	FOV	Slice Thick	Inter-space	NEX	TI	Pulse Sequence Options
Triple IR FSE		42	32	62	256	256	30-40/.75	5-8		1	BSP Auto	Gating, Sat-F, Seq, BSP, Zip 512, #RR 2, Trigger Delay Min
PC		Min full	20 FA	31.25	256	128	35/35	8	0	1		Gating Seq, Phase Diff. velocity 250
Post GAD												
2D Delayed Enhan-cement		Min	20 FA	25	224	160	35-38				Depen-dent on patient	Fast, IrP, ECG Gating, VPS 16-24, Trigger window 20, Trigger delay 300

(Continued)

Table 5-3						Cardiac MRI—*cont'd*							
Sequence 1.5	**TR**	**TE**	**ETL or FA**	**Band-width**	**F Matrix**	**Ph Matrix**	**FOV**	**Slice Thick**	**Inter-space**	**NEX**	**TI**	**Pulse Sequence Options**
Cor MRA aorta gated		Min	40 FA	62.5	512	256	40/.90	4		1		3-D Vasc TOF SPGR, Fast, ECG Gating, Zip 2, Asset
Sag MRA aorta Non-gated		Min	40 FA	62.5	320	192	36/.80	3		.75	32 loc/slab	3-D Vasc TOF SPGR, Zip 2, Asset, Fluoro multi-phase, 2 phases, auto-subtract

FOV is dependent on patient's size. The Zoom gradient should be used when available.
Make sure volume shim is placed directly over the heart and checked in all 3 planes.
Duplicate FIESTA for all cine, i.e., short axis, long axis, 2, 3, and 4 chamber acquisitions. BSP stands for blood suppression.
Arrhythmia rejection window = 20, Number of phases reconstruction = 20,
VENC Aorta 200-250cm/sec, PA 150-200 cm/sec.
Adjust the TI (inversion time) to maximize nullification of the myocardium on delayed enhancement.
Suggest a 10 second scan delay for gated MRA.
TRF (Tailor Radio-Frequency) should be used with all FSE sequence to increase # of slices per TR.

Sequence 1.5	TR	TE	ETL or FA	Band-width	F Matrix	Ph Matrix	FOV	Slice Thick	Inter-space	NEX	TI	Pulse Sequence Options
Post GAD												

Table 5-4 Site Protocol: Cardiac MRI

MRI OF THE BRACHIAL PLEXUS

Scan Considerations

- The brachial plexus is the network of nerves and fibers running from the spine, just above the fifth cervical vertebra to below the first thoracic vertebrae (C5-T1). The roots begin to divide into three primary cords posterior to the clavicle and travel laterally and inferiorly to below the axilla, where they again divide into five terminal branches. The branchial plexus provides stimulation for the muscles of the shoulder and upper extremities.
- Refer to all safety-related parameters discussed in the front matter at the beginning of the book (p. xiv-xix).
- As the SAR (specific absorption rate) increases, the patient's body temperature will also increase, particularly at 3T. It is important to monitor the SAR for the patient safely as well as to prevent scanning interruption.

Coils

- A multi-channel vender-specific neurovascular coil is recommended.
- All multi-channel coils produce excessive signal adjacent to the coil. This can be compensated for by using vendor-specific options, i.e., GE uses SCIC or PURE, to provide uniform signal intensity.

Pulse Sequences

- T1 and 1 FLAIR imaging is used to best identify anatomical structure, and T2 fat saturation provide detailed evidence of pathology.

- On T1 sequences, the nerves and vasculature of the brachial pelvis are seen as dark or hypo-intense signal surrounded by bright fat.
- T2 sequences, fat saturation, and/or STIR are performed to enhance abnormal fluid or pathology from trauma, fibrous bands, tumor, or infections.

Options

- IDEAL (GE), a fat/water separation technique (previously called 3 point Dixon technique), when used, gives uniform fat or water elimination. The brachial plexus can be challenging to scan because of the variations in anatomy that includes the base of the brain, cervical spine, thoracic spine, and shoulders. These variations often make it difficult to obtain uniform fat saturation. New vendor-specific sequences, i.e., IDEAL (GE) eliminate fat and water and provide a fat, water, in and out of phase image, all in one acquisition. IDEAL is used with T1, T2, and SPGR.
- Fat saturation options and terminology is vendor-specific. For GE systems, use "fat classic" for fat saturation with enhanced pathologic detail.
- Superior and inferior saturation bands help to compensate for vascular pulsation. An anterior saturation band should not be used because it will interfere with the brachial plexus anatomy.
- Flow compensation or gradient nulling should be used on T2 images to help compensate for vascular motion.

Imaging of the Brachial Plexus

Acquire a three-plane pilot per site specifications.

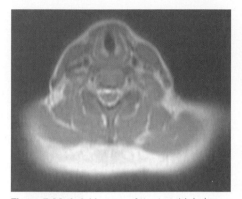

Figure 5-36 Axial Image of the brachial plexus

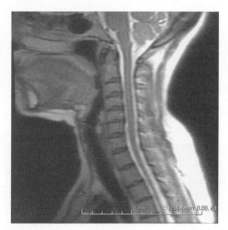

Figure 5-37 Sagittal image of the brachial plexus

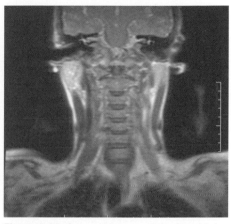

Figure 5-38 Coronal image of the brachial plexus

TIP: Avoid using anterior saturation bands during this study.

COIL: Multi-channel vendor-specific neurovascular coil
POSITION: Supine, head first
LANDMARK: Jugular notch of the sternum
IMMOBILIZATION: Instruct the patient to minimize swallowing and avoid heavy breathing. Secure the head to prevent rotation. Prevent the body from touching the sides of the magnet by using sponges or sheets.

Acquisition of Coronal Images

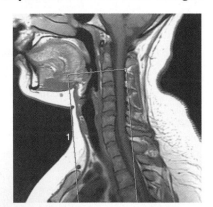

Figure 5-39 Sagittal image with coronal location

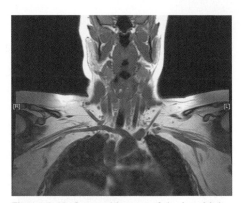

Figure 5-40 Coronal image of the brachial plexus

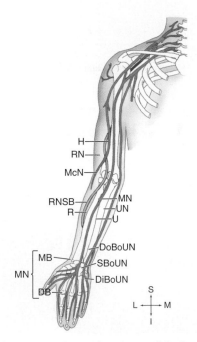

Figure 5-41 Coronal anatomy of the brachial plexus

SLICE ACQUISITION: Anterior to posterior
SLICE ALIGNMENT: Parallel to spine
ANATOMIC COVERAGE: Anterior neck wall through the posterior spinal cord, bilaterally to include coracoid processes

TIP: Bilateral images for comparison, especially in the coronal plane, are often acquired routinely regardless of the affected side.

KEY : **DB**, digital branch; **DiBoUN**, digital branch of ulnar nerve; **DoBoUN**, dorsal branch of ulnar nerve; **H**, humerus; **MB**, muscular branch; **McN**, musculocutaneous nerve; **MN**, median nerve; **R**, radius; **RN**, radial nerve; **RNSB**, radial nerve (superficial branch); **SBoUN**, superficial branch of ulnar nerve; **U**, ulna; **UN**, ulnar nerve.

Acquisition of Axial Images

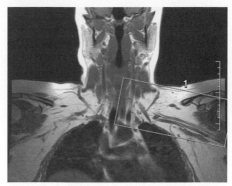

Figure 5-42 Coronal image with axial location

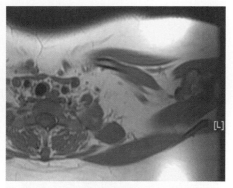

Figure 5-43 Axial image of the brachial plexus

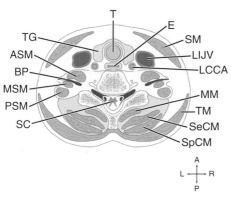

Figure 5-44 Axial anatomy of the brachial plexus

SLICE ACQUISITION: Superior to inferior

SLICE ALIGNMENT: Angle slices to be parallel with the brachial plexus

ANATOMIC COVERAGE: Anterior neck wall through posterior spinal cord, bilaterally to include the coracoid processes

KEY: **ASM**, anterior scalene muscle; **BP**, brachial plexus; **E**, esophagus; **LIJV**, left internal jugular vein; **LCCA**, left common carotid artery; **MM**, multifidus muscle; **MSM**, middle scalene muscle; **PSM**, posterior scalene muscle; **SM**, sternocleidomastoid muscle; **SeCM**, semispinalis capitis muscle; **SpCM**, splenius capitis muscle; **SC**, spinal cord; **T**, trachea; **TM**, trapezius muscle; **TG**, thyroid gland.

Acquisition of Sagittal Images

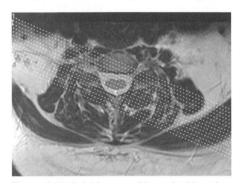

Figure 5-45 Axial image with sagittal location

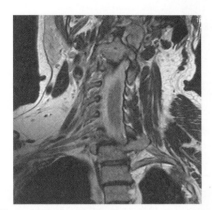

Figure 5-46 Sagittal image of the brachial plexus

SLICE ACQUISITION: Oblique anterior to posterior
SLICE ALIGNMENT: Angle slices to be perpendicular to the brachial plexus
ANATOMIC COVERAGE: C3 through T2

TIP: Minimize swallowing and heavy breathing

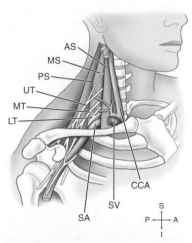

Figure 5-47 Sagittal anatomy of the brachial plexus

KEY: **AS**, anterior scalene; **CCA**, common carotid artery; **LT**, lower trunk; **MT**, middle trunk; **MS**, middle scalene; **PS**, posterior scalene; **SV**, subclavian vein; **SA**, subclavian artery; **UT**, upper trunk.

Table 5-5 MRI of the Brachial Plexus

Sequence 1.5	TR	TE	ETL or FA	Band-width	F Matrix	Ph Matrix	FOV	Slice Thick	Inter-space	NEX	TI	Pulse Sequence Options
Cor T1 FSE	600	Min	4	35.71	256	224	24/24	4	.5	4		Sat S-I, TRF, NPW
Cor STIR	4000	68	17	41.67	256	224	24/24	4	.5	3	110	FC, Seq, NPW
Ax T1 FSE	625	Min	3	35.71	256	224	20/20	4	0	2		Sat S-I, NPW
Ax T2 FRFSE FS	3500	85	27	41.67	320	224	20/20	4	0	4		Sat S-I, F, FC, NPW
Sag Obl T2 FRFSE	3500	85	18 ETL	41.67	448	224	24	2.2	1	4		FRFSE, sat I, FC, TRF, NPW
Post GAD												
Cor T1 FSE FS	600	Min	4	41.67	256	224	24/24	4	.5	4		Sat S-I, F, NPW
Ax T1 FSE	625	Min	3	41.67	256	224	20/20	4	0	2		Sat S-I, NPW

(Continued)

Table 5-5					MRI of the Brachial Plexus—*cont'd*								

Sequence 3T	TR	TE	ETL or FA	Band-width	F Matrix	Ph Matrix	FOV	Slice Thick	Inter-space	NEX	TI	Pulse Sequence Options
Cor T1 Flair	3000	22	8	41.67	448	224	24/24	4	0	2	Auto	Sat S-I, NPW
Cor STIR	4500	68	19	50	320	224	24/24	4	.5	3	170	FC, Seq, NPW
Ax T1 FSE	1100	Min	4	41.67	256	224	18/18	4	0	2		Sat S-I, NPW
Ax T2 FRFSE FS	3200	85	17	50	288	224	18/18	4	0	4		Sat S-I, FC, NPW
Sag Obl. T2 FRFSE	4000	110	21	50	416	224	24/24	3	.5	4		Sat S-I, FC, NPW
Post GAD												
Cor T1 FSE FS	1000	Min	4	41.67	448	224	24/24	4	.5	2		Sat S-I, F, NPW
Ax T1 FSE	1100	Min	4 ETL	41.67	448	224	18/18	4	0	2		Sat S-I, NPW

Adjust FOV depending on patient's size
T1 FSE ETL 4 of lower
TRF (Tailor Radio-Frequency) should be used with all FSE sequence to increase # of slices per TR
Use NPW when possibility of anatomy wrapping (No Phase Wrap)
When Fat saturation is ineffective use STIR or IDEAL when available (see grab bag for parameters)

Sequence 1.5	TR	TE	ETL or FA	Band-width	F Matrix	Ph Matrix	FOV	Slice Thick	Inter-space	NEX	TI	Pulse Sequence Options
Post GAD												

Table 5-6 Site Protocol: MRI of the Brachial Plexus

(Continued)

Table 5-6   Site Protocol: MRI of the Brachial Plexus—*cont'd*

Sequence 3T	TR	TE	ETL or FA	Band-width	F Matrix	Ph Matrix	FOV	Slice Thick	Inter-space	NEX	TI	Pulse Sequence Options
Post GAD												

MRI of the Abdomen and Pelvis

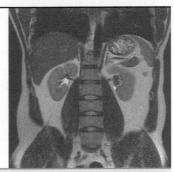

CHAPTER OUTLINE

MRI OF THE ABDOMEN AND PELVIS— CONSIDERATIONS

Scan Considerations

Refer to all vendor-specific safety parameters.

Ensure that the patient empties their bladder before scanning.

Patients should have an IV placed in the antecubital fossa prior to positioning when contrast is indicated. A 20-gauge angiocath is preferred. A power injector should be used for all abdominal MRI and MRA imaging for most effective contrast enhancement. For abdominal MRI and MRA, an injection rate of 1.5-2.0 cc/sec is suggested.

There are several types of contrasts used for imaging the abdomen and pelvis. Gadolinium-based contrast agent (GCBA) dosing is based on the patient's weight, and the manufactures dosing guidelines should be followed. The weight-based approach of 0.1 mmol/kg (0.2 mL/kg) followed by 20-30 mL of saline is recommended for extracellular contrast.

All contrast imaging should have pre contrast sequences prior to injection. Precontrast scans are multi-purpose.
• They allow for assessment of adequate anatomical coverage.
• They permit image review for asset artifacts in the FOV.
• They serve as a MASK for subsequent contrast sequences.

It is important to document the patient's contrast dose, flow rate and contrast agent used during the procedure, for the radiologist who will be interpreting the MR scan.

Secretin is a medication that enhances visualization of the pancreatic duct. A slow IV injection of 1 U/kg of secretin is given and a MRCP is performed immediately after the injection and several times post injection through the pancreatic duct until it is properly visualized.

Because of respiratory motion, breath-hold sequences are essential in abdominal MRI and MRA imaging. A respiratory bellows should be placed on the patient prior to positioning the patient in the coil. The respiratory bellows is used to monitor the patient's breathing pattern as well as to monitor their ability to follow breath-hold direction. Before positioning the patient on the table make sure you explain the importance of holding their breath. Breath hold sequences can be acquired either on inspiration or expiration but must be consistent.

Dielectric artifacts impact MRI studies by causing an increase in inhomogeneity. Dielectric effects are caused by local eddy currents due to the increased conductivity of body tissue. This effect is particularly prominent in 3T body imaging. There is shading, or a drop off of signal in the area being imaged. This effect is exaggerated when the patient has ascites. The dielectric effect in muscle is worse than that of fatty tissue. This inhomogeneity artifact can limit the scans diagnostic capabilities. Most vendors provide a dielectric pad, which should be placed on the patient's abdomen or pelvis before positioning the coil. Although the pad does not eliminate shading, it can effectively compensate for it. At 3T when the artifact limits the scan quality, the patient should be scanned on a 1.5T system.

Coils

A multi channel vendor specific array coil should be used for abdominal and pelvic imaging when available. A multi-channel cardiac coil can also be used particularly for the MRA of the renal arteries, MRCP, prostate and uterus. Configuration of the coils is dependent on the area of the abdomen and pelvis being scanned.

Pulse Sequences

Breath-hold T1 SPGR and T2 SSFSE can be acquired in 20 seconds or less.

Breath-hold T1 SPGR exhibits T1 contrast and best identifies anatomical structures. Dual SPGR In phase (2.2 TE) and Out of phase (4.4 TE) can help identify pancreatic and adrenal pathology. Fat saturation can be helpful in this pulse sequence to decrease bright fat signal seen on T1 imaging.

Breath-hold T2 SSFSE or FSE sequences best visualizes T2 contrast of the liver, pancreas, bile ducts, and kidneys. These sequences best delineate pathology of the structures. Fat saturation is used to further demonstrate pathology when fat is present.

FIESTA (Fast Imaging Employing Steady State Acquisition) is a sequence that identifies bright fluid and vessels in the abdomen without contrast. It is a non–breath-hold sequence, which can be acquired in the axial and coronal plane in approximately one minute each. It is an effective localizer for a MRCP and phase-contrast imaging of the portal vein, as well as defining the vascular structures of the abdomen and pelvis.

The MRCP uses a T2 FRFSE and SSFSE (high TR and TE) with fat saturation, to examine the biliary system in patients with possible biliary obstruction, stones. A 2D or 3D volume is acquired at the level of the common bile duct and head of the pancreas. This produces an image with heavily suppressed background and bright fluid.

3D LAVA is a high-resolution, dynamic, multi-phase T1 SPGR image with saturated fat. This contrast-enhanced sequence can identify the arterial, venous, and equilibrium phases of the liver and abdominal structures, as well as blood vessels. A dynamic LAVA precontrast scan is initially preformed and used as the MASK for increased contrast enhancement.

DWI imaging is performed on the liver with b-values of 50, 250, and 500 and higher. It is used for increased visualization and detection of the number of lesions present as well as to help to characterize the type of lesions present.

Gradient echo, susceptibility-weighted imaging sequences, is especially useful to demonstrate iron deposition in the liver (hemochromatosis).

Options

In parallel imaging (GE Asset), a reduced dataset in the phase encoding direction(s) of k-space is acquired to shorten the acquisition time by combining the signal of several coil arrays. A low-resolution, fully Fourier-encoded reference image (GE asset calibration scan) is required for sensitivity assessment. Asset is important in abdominal MRI and MRA because breath-hold imaging is necessary. Asset imaging cuts the scan time in half but needs a calibration scan to do so. Prescribe a calibration scan for each coil selected. Prescribe the asset scan superiorly and inferiorly at least four centimeters above and below the area of interest, to help avoid asset directional artifacts. A breath-hold calibration scan should be acquired in a single breath-hold acquisition.

All multi-channel coils produce excessive signal adjacent to the coil. This can be compensated for by using vendor-specific options, i.e., GE uses SCIC or PURE, to provide uniform signal intensity. When PURE is used a calibration scan is necessary.

Flouro trigger is an option that is used with dynamic imaging to follow the contrast as it enters the abdominal aorta. Contrast is injected with a power injector and the contrast is followed from the heart to the pulmonary arteries, to the aorta. When the contrast is detected entering the superior abdominal aorta, the post-contrast phase begins. Three post-contrast phases are acquired, each in a single breath hold of about 20 seconds.

The precontrast scan is used as a MASK for the subsequent dynamic contrast scans.

Saturation bands can be used on all pulse sequences. A Superior (S) and Inferior (I) saturation (Sat) bands can be used to help compensate for vascular pulsation and Anterior (A) saturation (Sat) can help to compensate for abdominal wall motion.

Fat saturation (FS) options and terminology are vendor specific. For GE systems use "fat classic" for fat saturation with enhanced anatomical detail. SPECIAL is a fat suppression technique used with 3D LAVA.

Flow compensation (FC) or gradient nulling should be used with T2 imaging to help compensate for vascular motion.

Scan Considerations for the Pelvis

When scanning the female pelvis, the anatomy of concern is the uterus, ovaries, and related structures. T2 images are performed in sagittal, and long and short axes of the uterus. Short axis is the coronal plane and the long axis is the axial plane of the uterus.

When scanning the male pelvis, the anatomy of concern is the prostate, seminal vesicles, neural bundles, and related structures. The prostate is often imaged with an endorectal coil, in conjunction with the torso or cardiac coil. The endorectal coil is placed in the patient's rectum and 50-70 cc of air is injected into the coil to keep it securely in place. For the male pelvis,

T2 imaging in all three planes is performed. T1 gradient echo imaging should be performed to identify residual blood, particularly after a prostate biopsy.

Scan Considerations for a Runoff of the Abdomen and Lower Extremities

MRAs or runoffs can be performed with 0.2–0.3 mmol/kg (0.4-0.6 mL/kg) of contrast agents that are FDA approved for multiple dosing (see contrast section). An injection rate of 1.5-2 cc/sec is suggested.

For TRICKS, an injection rate of 1.5 cc/sec is suggested. For a TRICKS sequence, a temporal resolution of approximately 7-10 sec should be used for claudication. Reduce temporal resolution to 3-6 seconds when ulceration of the lower limb is present to avoid venous contamination of surrounding tissue.

When scanning a runoff, a multi-station MRA of the abdomen, pelvis, and lower extremity, there are several coil considerations.

On a 1.5T scanner, a PV (peripheral vascular) coil can be used to scan the patient's vessels in their entirety, from top to bottom. When a PV coil is not available, the CTL coil can also be used at 1.5T or 3T.

A TRICKS (Time Resolved Imaging Contrast Kinetics) scan of the lower station, from the knees down is initially performed (first injection) and then a multi-station runoff, abdomen-pelvis, thighs, and lower leg (second injection), which follows the contrast from top to bottom.

When a CTL spine coil is used, the patient's lower legs should be positioned at the top station. The patient is positioned on the coil supine, feet first, and a TRICKS scan of the lower legs is performed. An additional 2-station runoff is acquired using the mid and lower portions of the coil. The patient's position on the coil must be considered and adjusted for proper coverage.

Place a sponge between the patient's legs and secure with sheets.

A noncontrast scan should always be performed at all stations to use as a MASK for increased tissue suppression and contrast enhancement.

It is recommended when scanning a runoff that thigh compression is used to decrease venous contamination. The use of thigh cuffs with long extension tubing, which can be inflated before the mask acquisition, will help to delay venous contamination (see Figures 4-87 through 4-89).

MRI OF THE ABDOMEN—KIDNEYS

Acquire three-plane pilot of the abdomen and pelvis per site specifications.

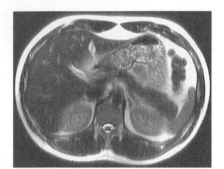

Figure 6-1 Axial abdomen and pelvis

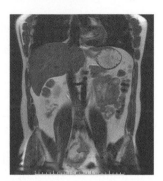

Figure 6-2 Coronal abdomen and pelvis

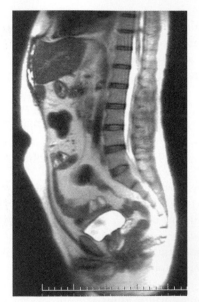

Figure 6-3 Sagittal abdomen and pelvis

COIL: Multi-channel or 12-channel torso array or multi-channel cardiac coil

SPECIAL CONSIDERATIONS: Position respiratory bellows on the patient before starting the scan at the level of the diaphragm. Position a diaelectric pad on the abdomen to help suppress shading artifacts.

POSITION: Supine, feet first, with coil covering diaphragm to iliac crest

Place patient's arms over the head or elevated on cushions away from the body.

LANDMARK: Midline, 4 inches above the iliac crest.

IMMOBILIZATION: Place a cushion under the patient's knees.

Prevent the body from touching the sides of the magnet by using sponges or sheets.

Acquisition of Coronal Images of the Abdomen

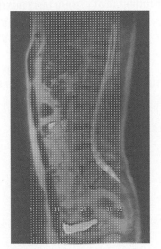

Figure 6-4 Sagittal image of the abdomen with coronal locations

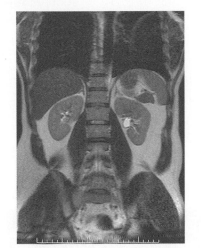

Figure 6-5 Coronal image of the abdomen

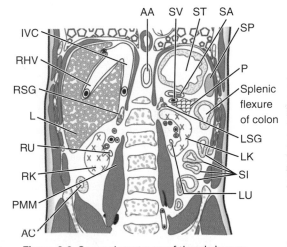

Figure 6-6 Coronal anatomy of the abdomen

SLICE ACQUISITION: Anterior to posterior
SLICE ALIGNMENT: Parallel to spine
ANATOMIC COVERAGE: From diaphragm to the pubis

KEY: **AA**, abdominal aorta; **AC**, ascending colon; **IVC**, inferior vena cava; **L**, liver; **LK**, left kidney; **LSG**, left suprarenal gland; **LU**, left ureter; **P**, pancreas; **PMM**, psoas major muscle; **RHV**, right hepatic vein; **RK**, right kidney; **RSG**, right suprarenal gland; **RU**, right ureter; **SA**, splenic artery; **SI**, small intestine; **SP**, spleen; **ST**, stomach; **SV**, splenic vein.

TIP: Practice breath-holds with the patient before starting the examination to ensure the patient's ability to hold their breath for an adequate time to ensure that all images are acquired at the same level of inspiration or expiration.

Acquisition of Axial Images of the Abdomen

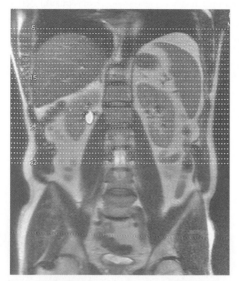

Figure 6-7 Coronal image of the abdomen with axial locations

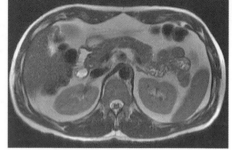

Figure 6-8 Axial image of the abdomen

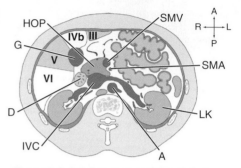

Figure 6-9 Axial anatomy of the abdomen

KEY: **A**, aorta; **D**, duodenum; **G**, gallbladder; **HOP**, head of pancreas; **IVC**, inferior vena cava; **LK**, left kidney; **SMA**, superior mesenteric artery; **SMV**, superior mesenteric vein.

SLICE ACQUISITION: Superior to inferior
SLICE ALIGNMENT: Straight; no angulation of slices is necessary.
ANATOMIC COVERAGE: From diaphragm to iliac crest

Acquisition of the Axial 3-D LAVA Images of the Abdomen

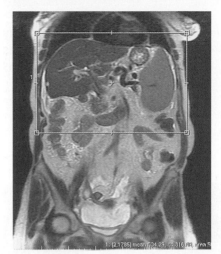

Figure 6-10 Coronal image of the abdomen with axial locations

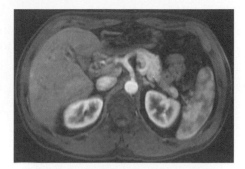

Figure 6-11 Axial image of the abdomen

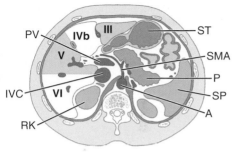

Figure 6-12 Axial anatomy of the abdomen

KEY: **A**, aorta; **IVC**, inferior vena cava; **P**, pancreas; **PV**, portal vein; **RK**, right kidney; **SMA**, superior mesenteric artery; **SP**, spleen; **ST**, stomach.

SLICE ACQUISITION: Superior to inferior
SLICE ALIGNMENT: Straight; no angulation of slices is necessary.
ANATOMIC COVERAGE: From diaphragm to the lower poles of the kidneys

TIP: Inform the patient that at this point he or she will be receiving a contrast injection. Instruct the patient to hold perfectly still and follow breathing instructions.

Acquisition of the Coronal 3-D Delayed Enhanced Images of the Abdomen and Pelvis

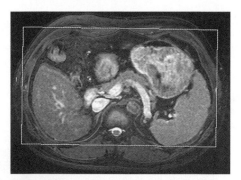

Figure 6-13 Axial image of the abdomen with coronal locations

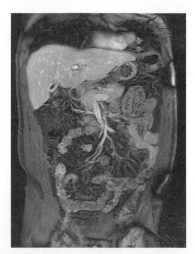

Figure 6-14 Coronal LAVA of the abdomen

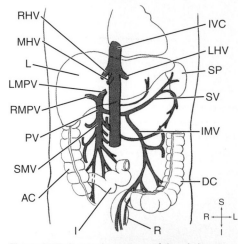

Figure 6-15 Coronal anatomy of the abdomen

SLICE ACQUISITION: Anterior to posterior
SLICE ALIGNMENT: Straight; no angulation of slices is necessary.
ANATOMIC COVERAGE: From anterior liver through the posterior kidneys

TIP: Reinforce the importance of holding perfectly still and following the breathing instructions.

KEY: **AC**, ascending colon; **DC**, descending colon; **I**, ileum; **IMV**, inferior mesenteric vein; **IVC**, inferior vena cava; **L**, liver; **LHV**, left hepatic vein; **LMPV**, left main portal vein; **MHV**, middle hepatic vein; **PV**, portal vein; **R**, rectum; **RHV**, right hepatic vein; **RMPV**, right main portal vein; **SMV**, superior mesenteric vein; **SP**, spleen; **SV**, splenic vein.

Table 6-1 MRI of the Abdomen

Sequence 1.5	TR	TE	ETL or FA	Band-width	F Matrix	Ph Matrix	FOV	Slice Thick	Inter-space	NEX	TI	Pulse Sequence Options
Cor T2 SSSFE	Min	90	Min	62.50	384	224	48/.90	5.0	0	1		Asset, Sat S-I
Cor Fiesta	Min	Mach	70 FA	83.33	192	320	35/35	4.0	.4	1		Fast, seq
Ax Fiesta	Min	Mach	70 FA	83.33	224	320	38/.80	4.0	.4	1		Fast, seq, Sat Fat/Special
Ax Dual IP-OP	175		90 FA	62.50	256	224	40/.80	8.0	0	1	2 echos	Fast, Asset, Sat S-I, Zip 512
Ax T2 SSSFE	Min	90	90 FA	62.50	384	224	40/.80	8.0	0	1		Asset, Sat S-I
Post GAD												
Ax 3-D Lava C-+	Mach		12 FA	62.50	320	160	40/.90	4.4	0	1	66 loc/slab	Special, Zip 2, Zip 512, Fluoro, Multiphase

(Continued)

Table 6-1	MRI of the Abdomen—*cont'd*

Sequence 1.5	TR	TE	ETL or FA	Band-width	F Matrix	Ph Matrix	FOV	Slice Thick	Inter-space	NEX	TI	Pulse Sequence Options
Cor 3-D Lava	Mach		12 FA	62.50	320	192	48/.90	4.0	0	1	44 loc/ slab	Special, Zip 512, Zip 2
Portal vein PC	24		30 FA	15.63	256	192	25	5.0	0	2	Venc 30	Vas PC, FC, NPW

Sequence 3T	TR	TE	ETL or FA	Band-width	F Matrix	Ph Matrix	FOV	Slice Thick	Inter-space	NEX	TI	Pulse Sequence Options
Cor T2 SSSFE	Min	100	90 FA	83.33	384	224	48/.90	5.0	0	1		Asset, Sat S-I
Cor Fiesta	Min	Mach	45 FA	125	160	160	35/35	4.0	.4	1		Fast, seq
Ax Fiesta	Min	Mach	45 FA	125	160	160	38/.80	4.0	.4	1		Fast, seq, Sat Fat/Special
Ax Dual IP	140	IP	80 FA	83.33	256	192	40/.80	8.0	0	1		Fast, Asset, Sat S-I, Zip 512

Table 6-1 MRI of the Abdomen—*cont'd*

Sequence 3T	TR	TE	ETL or FA	Band-width	F Matrix	Ph Matrix	FOV	Slice Thick	Inter-space	NEX	TI	Pulse Sequence Options
Ax Dual OP	140	OP	80 FA	83.33	256	192	40/.80	8.0	0	1		Fast, Asset, Sat S-I, Zip 512
Ax T2 SSSFE	Min	100		83.33	448	192	40/.80	8.0	0	1		Asset, Sat S-I
Post GAD												
Ax 3D Lava C-+	Mach		12 FA	62.50	320	192	42/.90	4.4	0	1	66 loc/slab	Special, Zip 512, Zip 2, Fluoro, Multiphase
Cor 3D Lava	Mach		12 FA	62.50	320	192	48/.90	4.0	0	1	44 loc/slab	Special, Zip 512, Zip 2
Portal Vein PC	33		30 FA	32.50	256	192	25	5.0	0	2	Venc 30	Vas PC, FC, NPW

FOV and loc/slab are dependent on patient's size.

Make sure to keep the breath-hold sequences approximately 20 seconds. All sequences are breath hold except for the fiesta sequence.

Use a dielectric pad on the abdomen to suppress shading artifacts.

LAVA, 3 phases post contrast. A 3D dual echo should be substituted for 2D dual echo In and Out of phase when available.

Table 6-2 Site Protocol: MRI of the Abdomen

Sequence 1.5	TR	TE	ETL or FA	Band-width	F Matrix	Ph Matrix	FOV	Slice Thick	Inter-space	NEX	TI	Pulse Sequence Options
Post GAD												

Table 6-2   Site Protocol: MRI of the Abdomen —*cont'd*

Sequence 3T	TR	TE	ETL or FA	Band-width	F Matrix	Ph Matrix	FOV	Slice Thick	Inter-space	NEX	TI	Pulse Sequence Options
Post GAD												

MRI OF THE ABDOMEN—PORTAL VEIN

Follow the scan protocol for abdomen and kidneys, adding a sequence for the portal vein.

Acquisition of the Portal Vein

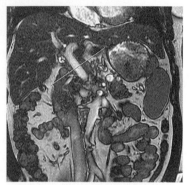

Figure 6-16 Coronal image of the abdomen with locations for the portal vein

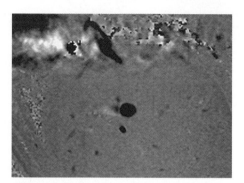

Figure 6-17 Anatomy of the portal system

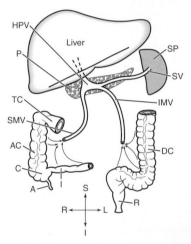

Figure 6-18 Image of the portal vein flow

SLICE ACQUISITION: Single slice angled through the portal vein

SLICE ALIGNMENT: Perpendicular to portal vein

ANATOMIC COVERAGE: Single slice through the portal vein; cross section portal vein and surrounding tissue.

TIP: This study is performed to assess flow or malignant invasion into the portal vein.

KEY: **A**, appendix; **AC**, ascending colon; **C**, cecum; **DC**, descending colon; **HPV**, hepatic portal vein; **I**, ileum; **IMV**, inferior mesenteric vein; **P**, pancreas; **R**, rectum; **SMV**, superior mesenteric vein; **SP**, spleen; **SV**, splenic vein; **TC**, transverse colon.

Table 6-3 Abdomen with EOVIST

Sequence 1.5	TR	TE	ETL or FA	Band-width	F Matrix	Ph Matrix	FOV	Slice Thick	Inter-space	NEX	TI	Pulse Sequence Options
Cor T2 SSSFE	Min	90		62.50	384	224	48/.90	5.0	0	1		Asset, Sat S-I
Ax Dual IP-OP	175				256	224	40/.80	8.0	0	1	2 echos	Fast, Asset, Zip 512
Post GAD												
Ax 3D Lava C-+	Mach		12 FA	62.50	320	160	40/.90	4.4	0	1	66 loc/ slab	Special, Zip 2, Zip 512, Fluoro, MP
Cor 3D Lava	Mach		12 FA	62.50	320	192	48/.90	4.0	0	1	44 loc/ slab	Special, Zip 2, Zip 512
Cor Fiesta	Min	Mach	70 FA	83.33	192	320	35/35	4.0	.4	1		Fast, Seq
Ax Fiesta	Min	Mach	70 FA	83.33	224	320	38/.80	4.0	.4	1		Fast, Seq, Sat Fat/Special
Ax T2 SSSFE	Min	90		62.50	384	224	40/.80	8.0	0	1		Asset, Sat S-I
Ax DWI EPI	Min	3525		62.50	160	128	40	8.0	0	2		B-value 50, 250, 500
Portal vein PC	24		30 FA	15.63	256	192	25	5.0	0	2	Venc 30	Vas PC, FC, NPW
Delayed Ax Lava	Mach		12 FA	62.50	320	160	40/.90	4.4	0	1	66 loc/ slab	Special, Zip 2, Zip 512

(Continued)

| Table 6-3 | Abdomen with EOVIST—*cont'd* |

Sequence 1.5	TR	TE	ETL or FA	Band-width	F Matrix	Ph Matrix	FOV	Slice Thick	Inter-space	NEX	TI	Pulse Sequence Options
Cor Lava	Mach		12 FA	62.50	320	192	48/.90	4.0	0	1	44 loc/ slab	Special, Zip 2, Zip 512
Cor 3D MRCP FRFSE				31.25	320	320	32/32	1.4	0	1	60-70 loc/ slab	Sat F, Zip 2, Asset, Respiratory Trigger

Sequence 3T	TR	TE	ETL or FA	Band-width	F Matrix	Ph Matrix	FOV	Slice Thick	Inter-space	NEX	TI	Pulse Sequence Options
Cor T2 SSSFE	Min	140		83.33	384	224	48/.90	5.0	0	1		SS, Fast, Asset, Sat S-I
Ax dual IP	140	IP	80 FA	83.33	384	192	40/.80	8.0	0	1		Fast, Asset, Zip 512
Ax dual OP	140	OP	80 FA	83.33	384	192	40/.80	8.0	0	1		Fast, Asset, Zip 512
Post GAD												
Ax 3D Lava C-+	Mach		12 FA	62.50	320	192	42/.90	4.4	0	1	66 loc/ slab	Special, Zip 512, Zip 2, Fluoro, MP

Sequence 3T	TR	TE	ETL or FA	Band-width	F Matrix	Ph Matrix	FOV	Slice Thick	Inter-space	NEX	TI	Pulse Sequence Options
Cor 3D Lava	Mach		12 FA	62.50	320	192	48/.90	4.0	0	1	44 loc/ slab	Special, Zip 512, Zip 2
Cor Fiesta	Min	Mach	45 FA	125	160	160	35/35	4.0	.4	1		Fast, Seq
Ax Fiesta	Min	Mach	45 FA	125	160	160	38/.80	4.0	.4	1		Fast, Seq, Sat Fat/ Special
Ax T2 SSSFE	Min	100		83.33	448	192	40/.80	8.0	0	1		Asset, sat S-I
Ax DWI EPI	Min	3525		62.50	160	128	40	8.0	0	2		B-value 50, 250, 500
Portal vein PC	33		30 FA	32.50	256	192	25	5.0	0	2	Venc 30	Vas PC, FC, NPW
Delayed Ax Lava	Mach		12 FA	83.33	320	192	48/.90	4.0	0	1	50 loc/ slab	Special, Zip 2 Zip 512, EDR
Cor 3D Lava	Mach		12FA	62.50	320	192	48/.90	4.0	0	1	44 loc/ slab	Special, Zip 512, Zip 2
Cor 3D MRCP FRFSE				31.25	320	320	30/30	1.4	0	1	60-70 loc/ slab	Sat F, Zip 2, Asset, Respiratory Trigger

Follow all abdomen tips above (6.1). Inject EOVIST and perform initial LAVA to visualize the arterial, venous, and equilibrium phases.
MP–Multiphase. Repeat the BH DWI three times with B-value 50, 250, and 500, each approximately 20 seconds.
Perform delayed single phase Ax 3D Lava and Cor at 20 minutes post EOVIST.
Mach–Machine-generated.

Table 6-4 Site Protocol: Abdomen with EOVIST

Sequence 1.5	TR	TE	ETL or FA	Band-width	F Matrix	Ph Matrix	FOV	Slice Thick	Inter-space	NEX	TI	Pulse Sequence Options
Post GAD												

Table 6-4	Site Protocol: Abdomen with EOVIST —*cont'd*											
Sequence 3T	TR	TE	ETL or FA	Band-width	F Matrix	Ph Matrix	FOV	Slice Thick	Inter-space	NEX	TI	Pulse Sequence Options
Post GAD												

MAGNETIC RESONANCE CHOLANGIOGRAPHIC PANCREATOGRAPHY

Acquire three-plane pilot of the abdomen per site specifications for MRCP.

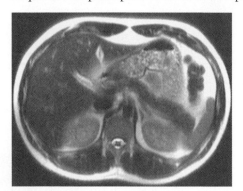

Figure 6-19 Axial abdomen

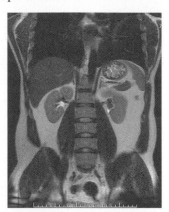

Figure 6-20 Coronal abdomen

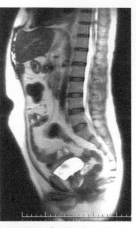

Figure 6-21 Sagittal abdomen

COIL: Multi-channel cardiac coil, multi-channel torso array

SPECIAL CONSIDERATIONS: Position respiratory bellows on the patient before starting the scan at the level of the diaphragm. Position a dielectric pad on the abdomen to help suppress shading artifacts (may also be used at 1.5T).

POSITION: Supine, feet first

LANDMARK: Midline, 4 inches above the iliac crest

IMMOBILIZATION: Place cushion under the patient's knees. Prevent body from touching the sides of the magnet by using sponges or sheets.

TIP: Patients should consume only clear fluids 2 hours before the examination

Acquisition of Coronal 3-D MRCP with Respiratory Trigger

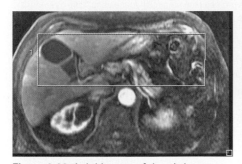

Figure 6-22 Axial image of the abdomen with coronal 3D locations

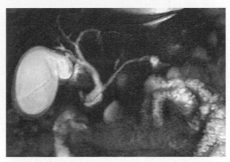

Figure 6-23 Coronal image of the biliary system

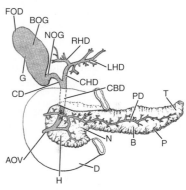

Figure 6-24 Coronal anatomy of the biliary system

SLICE ACQUISITION: Anterior to posterior

SPECIAL CONSIDERATIONS: Position respiratory bellows on the patient before starting the scan at the level of the diaphragm. Position a dielectric pad on the abdomen to help suppress shading artifacts.

SLICE ALIGNMENT: Straight, no angulation of slices

ANATOMIC COVERAGE: Gallbladder to aorta including head of pancreas

> *KEY:* **AOV**, ampulla of Vater; **B**, body; **BOG**, body of gallbladder; **CBD**, common bile duct; **CD**, cystic duct; **CHD**, common hepatic duct; **D**, duodenum; **FOD**, fundus of gallbladder; **G**, gallbladder; **H**, head; **LHD**, left hepatic duct; **N**, neck; **NOG**, neck of gallbladder; **P**, pancreas; **PD**, pancreatic duct; **RHD**, right hepatic duct; **T**, tail.

> *TIP:* Perform post-contrast when accompanying a contrast-enhanced study of the abdomen. This 3-D sequence may be reformatted to produce multiple planes through the biliary system.

Acquisition of Radial (Thick Slab) Images for MRCP

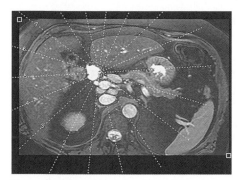

Figure 6-25 Axial image of the abdomen with multiple locations through the biliary system

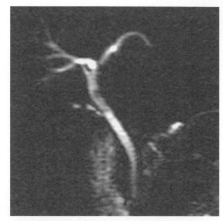

Figure 6-26 Image of the gallbladder and biliary ducts

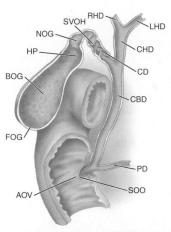

Figure 6-27 Anatomy of the gallbladder and biliary system

SLICE ACQUISITION: Multiple spoke-like slices through the gallbladder and ducts
SLICE ALIGNMENT: Align to structures of the gallbladder and biliary system
ANATOMIC COVERAGE: Anterior liver to kidneys

TIP: Be sure to include the head of the pancreas. If secretin is injected to enhance visualization of the pancreatic duct, scan every 3 minutes until desired visualization is achieved. Radiologist should select the most desirable MRCP image to be scanned over several minutes.

KEY: **AOV**, ampulla of Vater; **BOG**, body of gallbladder; **CBD**, common bile duct; **CD**, cystic duct; **CHD**, common hepatic duct; **FOG**, fundus of gallbladder; **HP**, Hartmann's pouch; **LHD**, left hepatic duct; **NOG**, neck of gallbladder; **PD**, pancreatic duct; **RHD**, right hepatic duct; **SOO**, sphincter of Oddi; **SVOH**, spiral valves of Hester.

Table 6-5 MRCP

Sequence 1.5	TR	TE	ETL or FA	Band-width	F Matrix	Ph Matrix	FOV	Slice Thick	Inter-space	NEX	TI	Pulse Sequence Options
Ax Fiesta	Min		70 FA	83.33	224	320	38/.80	4	.4	1		Fiesta, Fast, seq, Sat Fat/ Special
Cor Fiesta	Min		70 FA	83.33	192	320	35/35	4	.4	1		Seq, Sat F
3D cor MRCP FRFSE				31.25	320	320	32/32	1.4	0	1	60-70 loc/ slab	Sat F, RT, Zip 2, Asset, Respiratory Trigger
Radial MRCP SSFSE	6000	1300		31.25	480	256	32/32	40	0	1		Sat F
Opt Thin SSFSE MRCP		250		31.25	256	224	38	4	0	1		Sat F, Asset

(Continued)

Table 6-5 MRCP—*cont'd*

Sequence 3T	TR	TE	ETL or FA	Band-width	F Matrix	Ph Matrix	FOV	Slice Thick	Inter-space	NEX	TI	Pulse Sequence Options
Ax Fiesta	Min		45 FA	125	160	160	38/.80	4	.4	1		Fiesta, fast, seq, Sat Fat/ Special
cor Fiesta	Min		45 FA	125	160	160	35/35	4	.4	1		Seq, Sat F
3D cor MRCP FRFSE				31.25	320	320	30/30	1.4	0	1	60-70 loc/ slab	Sat F, Zip 2, Asset, Respiratory Trigger
Radial MRCP	6000	1300		31.25	480	256	30/30	40	0	1		Sat F
Opt Thin SSFSE MRCP		250		31.25	256	224	38	4	0	1		Sat F, Asset

FOV is dependent on patient's size.
Use a dielectric pad on the abdomen to suppress shading artifacts.
When contrast is administered scan the MRCP post gadolinium.
3D Respiratory Triggered MRCP can be reformatted post acquisition.
Radial (thick) 12 thick slices in a spoke like acquisition.

Table 6-6 Site Protocol: MRCP

Sequence 1.5	TR	TE	ETL or FA	Band-width	F Matrix	Ph Matrix	FOV	Slice Thick	Inter-space	NEX	TI	Pulse Sequence Options

Sequence 3T	TR	TE	ETL or FA	Band-width	F Matrix	Ph Matrix	FOV	Slice Thick	Inter-space	NEX	TI	Pulse Sequence Options

MRI OF THE ADRENAL GLANDS

Acquire three-plane pilot of the abdomen as per site protocol.

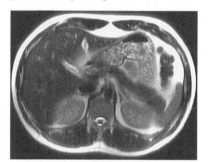

Figure 6-28 Axial abdomen

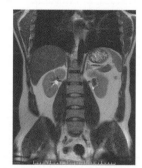

Figure 6-29 Coronal abdomen

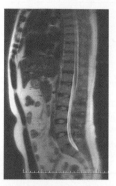

Figure 6-30 Sagittal abdomen

COIL: Multi-channel torso array or multi-channel cardiac coil

SPECIAL CONSIDERATIONS: Position respiratory bellows on the patient before starting the scan at the level of the diaphragm. Position a dielectric pad on the abdomen to help suppress shading artifacts; this pad may also be used for 1.5 T.

POSITION: Supine, feet first, with coil covering the diaphragm to the iliac crest. Place the patient's arms over the head or elevated on cushions away from the body.

LANDMARK: Midline, 4 inches above the iliac crest.

IMMOBILIZATION: Place a cushion under the patient's knees. Prevent the body from touching sides of the magnet by using sponges or sheets.

Acquisition of Axial Images of the Adrenals

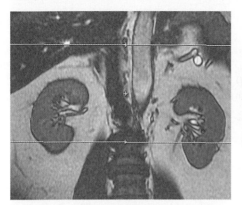

Figure 6-31 Coronal image of the abdomen with axial locations for the adrenal glands

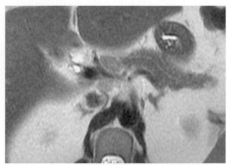

Figure 6-32 Axial image of the adrenal glands

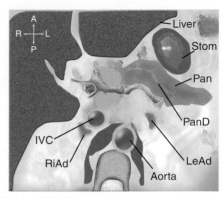

Figure 6-33 Axial anatomy of the adrenal glands

SLICE ACQUISITION: Superior to inferior

SLICE ALIGNMENT: Straight with no angulation of slices

ANATOMIC COVERAGE: From diaphragm to renal pelvis

KEY: IVC, inferior vena cava; **LeAd**, left adrenal; **Pan**, pancreas; **PanD**, pancreatic duct; **RiAd**, right adrenal; **Stom**, stomach.

TIP: Although multiple sequences with varying parameters are suggested in the accompanying table, anatomic coverage and slice placement for images in the axial plane are the same.

Acquisition of Coronal Images of the Adrenal Glands

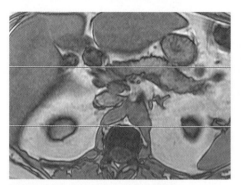

Figure 6-34 Axial image of the abdomen with coronal locations for the adrenal glands

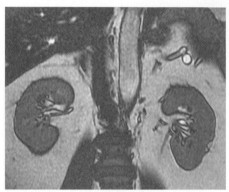

Figure 6-35 Coronal image of the adrenal glands

Figure 6-36 Coronal anatomy of the adrenal glands

KEY: **A**, aorta; **AG**, adrenal gland; **C**, cortex; **CT**, celiac trunk; **ISA**, inferior suprarenal artery; **IVC**, inferior vena cava; **K**, kidney; **M**, medulla; **MSA**, middle suprarenal artery; **RA**, renal artery; **RV**, renal vein; **SMA**, superior mesenteric artery.

SLICE ACQUISITION: Anterior to posterior

SLICE ALIGNMENT: Straight with no angulation of slices

ANATOMIC COVERAGE: From the body of the pancreas to the anterior aspect of the vertebral body

TIP: Dual SPGR, in- and out-of-phase imaging, can identify adenoma versus other adrenal pathology.

Table 6-7 Adrenal Glands

Sequence 1.5	TR	TE	ETL or FA	Band-width	F Matrix	Ph Matrix	FOV	Slice Thick	Inter-space	NEX	TI	Pulse Sequence Options
Cor T2 SSSFE	Min	90		62.50	384	224	36-42	5.0	0	1		Asset, Sat S-I
Ax dual IP-OP	225		75 FA	31.25	256	224	36-40/.80	5.0	0	1	2 echos	Fast, Asset, Zip 512
Cor Dual IP-OP	225		75 FA	31.25	320	224	36-42	5.0	0	1	2 echos	Fast, Asset, Zip 512
Cor Fiesta	Min		70 FA	83.33	192	320	35/35	4.0	.4	1		Fast, Seq
Ax T2 SSSFE	Min	90		62.50	384	224	40/.80	4.0	0	1		Asset, Sat S-I
Post GAD												
Ax Lava C-+	Mach		12 FA	62.50	320	192	42/.80	4.4	0	1	50 loc/ slab	Sat Special, Zip 2, Zip 512, Fluoro, Multiphase
Cor Lava	Mach		12 FA	62.50	320	192	48/.90	4.0	0	1	40 loc/ slab	Sat Special, Zip 2, Zip 512

(Continued)

| Table 6-7 | | | | | | | | | | | | Adrenal Glands—*cont'd* |

Sequence 3T	TR	TE	ETL or FA	Band-width	F Matrix	Ph Matrix	FOV	Slice Thick	Inter-space	NEX	TI	Pulse Sequence Options
Cor T2 SSSFE	Min	90		62.50	384	224	36-42	5.0	0	1		Asset, Sat S-I
Ax dual IP	140	IP	80 FA	62.50	256	192	40/.80	4.0	0	1		Fast, Asset, Zip 512
Ax dual OP	140	OP	80 FA	62.50	256	192	40/.80	4.0	0	1		Fast, Asset, Zip 512
Cor dual IP	225	IP	75 FA	31.25	320	224	36-42	4.0	0	1		Fast, Asset, Zip 512
Cor dual OP	225	OP	75 FA	31.25	320	224	36-42	4.0	0	1		Fast, Asset, Zip 512
Cor Fiesta	Min		45 FA	125	160	160	35/35	4.0	.4	1		Fast, Seq
Ax T2 SSSFE	Min	90		62.50	384	224	36-40 /.80	4.0	0	1		Asset, Sat S-I

Table 6-7 Adrenal Glands—*cont'd*

Sequence 3T	TR	TE	ETL or FA	Band-width	F Matrix	Ph Matrix	FOV	Slice Thick	Inter-space	NEX	TI	Pulse Sequence Options
Post GAD												
Ax Lava XV C-+	Mach		12 FA	83.33	320	192	42/.80	4.4	0	1	50 loc/slab	Sat Special, Zip 2, Zip 512, Fluoro, Multiphase
Cor Lava XV	Mach		12 FA	83.33	320	192	48/.90	4.0	0	1	40 loc/slab	Sat Special, Zip 2, Zip 512

Adjust FOV and loc/slab depending on patient's size. All sequences are breath hold except for the fiesta sequence.

In-phase TE 2.2 and Out-phase TE 4.4, 3D dual echo should be substituted for 2D dual echo In and Out of phase when available.

Use a dielectric pad on the abdomen to suppress shading artifacts.

Perform LAVA sequence when contrast is ordered.

Table 6-8 Site Protocol - Adrenal Glands

Sequence 1.5	TR	TE	ETL or FA	Band-width	F Matrix	Ph Matrix	FOV	Slice Thick	Inter-space	NEX	TI	Pulse Sequence Options
Post GAD												

Table 6-8	Site Protocol - Adrenal Glands—*cont'd*											
Sequence 3T	TR	TE	ETL or FA	Band-width	F Matrix	Ph Matrix	FOV	Slice Thick	Inter-space	NEX	TI	Pulse Sequence Options
Post GAD												

MRI OF THE FEMALE PELVIS—UTERUS

Acquire three-plane pilot per site specifications.

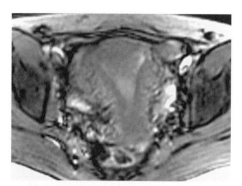

Figure 6-37 Axial image of the pelvis

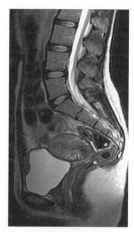

Figure 6-38 Sagittal image of the pelvis

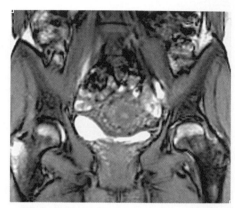

Figure 6-39 Coronal image of the pelvis

COIL: Multi-channel torso array or multi-channel cardiac coil

POSITION: Position the patient supine, feet first with coil covering iliac crest to proximal femurs.

LANDMARK: ASIS, midcoil

IMMOBILIZATION: Place hands on the chest or at the patient's side.

Prevent the body from touching the sides of the magnet by using sponges or sheets.

TIP: The primary purpose for this study is to examine the uterus, which will be referred to structurally in terms of short axis (anterior to posterior), and long axis (superior to inferior). Do not perform this examination during the patient's menses.

Acquisition of Sagittal Images of the Uterus

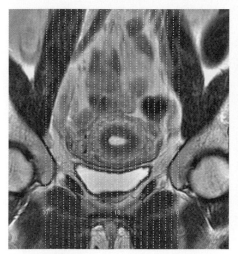

Figure 6-40 Coronal image of the pelvis with sagittal locations through the uterus

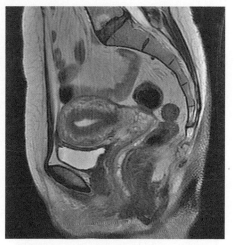

Figure 6-41 Sagittal image of the uterus

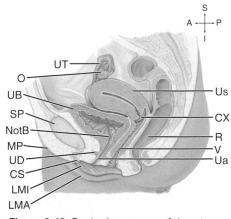

Figure 6-42 Sagittal anatomy of the uterus

KEY: **CS**, clitoris; **CX**, cervix; **LMA**, labia majora; **LMI**, labia minora; **MP**, mons pubis; **NotB**, neck of the bladder; **O**, ovary; **R**, rectum; **SP**, symphysis pubis; **Ua**, urethra; **UB**, urinary bladder; **UD**, urogenital diaphragm; **Us**, uterus; **UT**, uterine (fallopian) tube; **V**, vagina.

SLICE ACQUISITION: Left to right

SLICE ALIGNMENT: Straight sagittal, no angulation

ANATOMIC COVERAGE: Left to right acetabulum, ASIS to obturator foramen

TIP: Do not perform this examination during the patient's menses.

Acquisition of Coronal (Short-Axis) Images of the Uterus

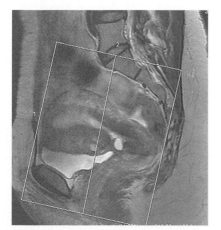

Figure 6-43 Sagittal image of the female pelvis with coronal (short-axis) locations

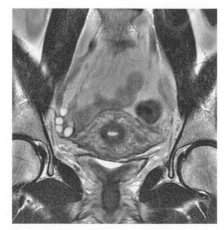

Figure 6-44 Coronal image of the female pelvis

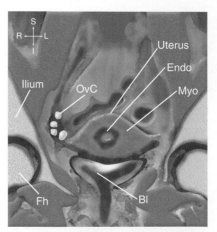

Figure 6-45 Coronal anatomy of the female pelvis

KEY: **Bl**, bladder; **Endo**, endometrium; **Fh**, femoral head; **Myo**, myometrium; **OvC**, ovarian cysts.

SLICE ACQUISITION: Anterior to posterior
SLICE ALIGNMENT: Perpendicular to the long axis of the uterus
ANATOMICAL COVERAGE: Pubis to anterior coccyx, to include the cervix and vagina

TIP: The position and size of the uterus vary greatly; cross-reference slice placement in all planes. If fibroids are present, perform coronal acquisition without angulation.

Acquisition of Axial (Long-Axis) Images of the Uterus

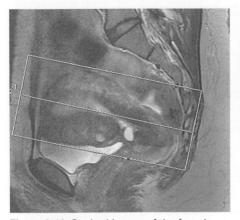

Figure 6-46 Sagittal image of the female pelvis with axial (long-axis) locations

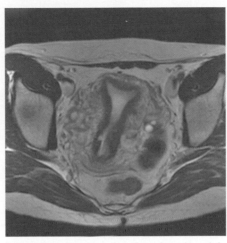

Figure 6-47 Axial image of the female pelvis

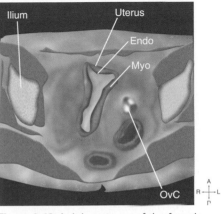

Figure 6-48 Axial anatomy of the female pelvis

SLICE ACQUISITION: Superior to inferior
SLICE ALIGNMENT: Parallel to long axis of uterus
ANATOMIC COVERAGE: Superior to inferior margins covering long axis of the uterus

KEY: **Endo**, endometrium; **Myo**, myometrium; **OvC**, ovarian cysts.

TIP: If fibroids are present, perform axial acquisition without angulation.

Table 6-9													
Female Pelvis and Uterus													
Sequence 1.5	**TR**	**TE**	**ETL or FA**	**Band-width**	**F Matrix**	**Ph Matrix**	**FOV**	**Slice Thick**	**Inter-space**	**NEX**	**TI**	**Pulse Sequence Options**
Ax T2 SSSFE	Min	90		62.50	384	224	40/.80	8.0	0	1		Asset, Sat S-I
Sag T2 FRFSE	5000	102	20	41.67	320	224	20-26	4.0	.5	4		Sat A-S, FC, NPW, Zip 512
Cor T2 FRFSE	5000	102	20	41.67	320	224	20-26	5.0	.5	2		Sat A-S, FC, NPW, Zip 512
Ax T2 FRFSE	5000	102	20	41.67	320	224	20-26	5.0	.5	2		Sat A-S, FC, NPW, Zip 512
Post GAD												
Ax Lava	Mach		12 FA	62.50	320	160	40/.90	4.4	0	1	66 loc/ slab	Sat Special, Zip 2, Zip 512, Fluoro, Multiphase
Cor FGRE	300	IP	80 FA	31.25	256	192	20/26	4.0	.5	1		Sat F, Zip 512

Table 6-9		Female Pelvis and Uterus—*cont'd*										
Sequence 3T	TR	TE	ETL or FA	Band-width	F Matrix	Ph Matrix	FOV	Slice Thick	Inter-space	NEX	TI	Pulse Sequence Options
Ax T2 SSSFE	Min	90		83.33	384	224	40/.80	8.0	0	1		Asset, Sat S-I
Sag T2 FRFSE	5000	120	24	62.50	320	224	20-26	4.0	.5	2		Sat A-S, FC, NPW, Zip 512
Cor T2 FRFSE	5000	120	24	62.50	320	224	20-26	4.0	.5	2		Sat A-S, FC, NPW, Zip 512
Ax T2 FRFSE	5000	120	24	62.50	320	224	20-26	4.0	.5	4		Sat A-S, FC, NPW, Zip 512
Post GAD												
Ax Lava	Mach		12 FA	83.33	320	192	30/.90	4.4	0	1	66 loc/ slab	Sat Special, Zip 2, Zip 512, Fluoro, Multiphase
Cor FGRE	300	IP	80 FA	41.67	256	256	20/26	4.0	0	1		Sat F, Zip 512

Adjust FOV and loc/slab depending on patient's size.
Ax T2 SSFSE from the kidneys to the pubis.
Use a dielectric pad on the pelvis to suppress shading artifacts.
TRF (Tailor Radio-Frequency) should be used with all FSE sequence to increase # of slices per TR.
Perform LAVA sequence when contrast is ordered.

Table 6-10 Site Protocol: Female Pelvis and Uterus

Sequence 1.5	TR	TE	ETL or FA	Band-width	F Matrix	Ph Matrix	FOV	Slice Thick	Inter-space	NEX	TI	Pulse Sequence Options
Post GAD												

Sequence 3T	TR	TE	ETL or FA	Band-width	F Matrix	Ph Matrix	FOV	Slice Thick	Inter-space	NEX	TI	Pulse Sequence Options
Post GAD												

Scan Consideration for MRI of the Fetus

Ultrasound is the primary modality used to evaluate the fetus. When an abnormal finding is suggested which needs further evaluation or clarification MRI can be performed. MRI can image the fetal brain, spinal canal, neck, chest, abdomen and pelvis using very fast T2 single shot imaging sequences. Assessment of brain abnormalities includes hydrocephalus, agenesis of the corpus callosum, cerebral mylination and posterior fossa masses. It can also demonstrate spinal abnormalities such as masses and spina bifida, congenital diaphragmatic hernia, bronchial atresia and airway compression of the chest. Complicated abdominal masses as well as kidney and urinary tract abnormalities are also visualized. Patients are also imaged when abnormal serum markers or chromosomal anomalies are identified. MRI is also very useful when appendicitis or placenta accreta in the mother are suspected.

Sedation is not necessary since fast sequences can be performed in seconds. The patient should be told to empty her bladder prior to performing the exam.

An informed consent should be obtained prior to scanning.

The importance of holding still should be stressed with the mother. She can be placed supine or on her side making her as comfortable as possible. A multi-channel torso coil is used to perform the exam.

MRI uses higher-resolution SSFSE and FIESTA ultra fast imaging which can detect subtle defects. These T2 sequences provide bright fluid signal surrounding the fetus, in vessels and in the ventricles of the brain. DWI of the fetal brain is added when stroke or mass is suspected. T1 FSPRG can be performed when T1 contrast is necessary, i.e. characterizing hemorrhage in the fetus.

The fetus is imaged in the axial, sagittal and coronal oblique projection anatomic to the fetus. The FOV should be large enough to avoid wrap on the scan. A radiologist is usually available during image acquisition to make sure the area of interest is being properly visualized.

Fetal MRI

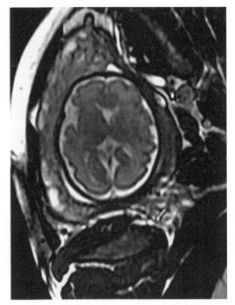

Figure 6-49 Axial image of the fetal brain

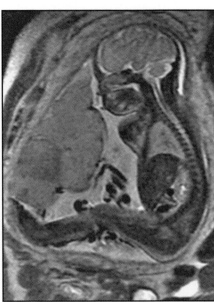

Figure 6-50 Sagittal image of the fetus

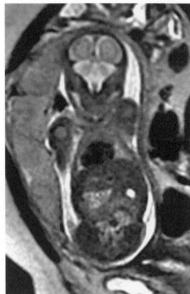

Figure 6-51 Coronal image of the fetus

COIL: Multi-channel torso
POSITION: Supine or decub, head first, cushion under or between knees
LANDMARK: Iliac crest

> ***TIP:*** The mother may eat cookies before scanning to reduce motion of the fetus.

MRI OF THE MALE PELVIS — PROSTATE

Acquire three-plane pilot per site specifications. Refer to table to acquire high-resolution sagittal locations before planning prostate scans.

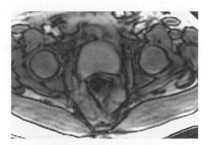

Figure 6-52 Axial image of the pelvis

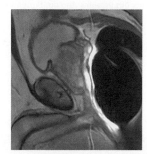

Figure 6-53 Sagittal image of the pelvis

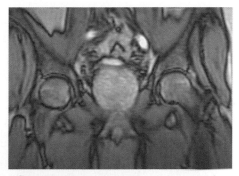

Figure 6-54 Coronal image of the pelvis

COIL: A disposable vendor-specific endo-rectal coil is suggested. Follow manufacturer's guidelines for use. It may be used in conjunction with the multi-channel cardiac or torso array. Coils can be integrated or used independently during scanning. The endo-rectal coil should be inflated with 50 to 70 mL of air, bearing in mind patient comfort. Do not use an endo-rectal coil if the patient has had a prostatectomy.

POSITION: Supine, feet first, legs flat

LANDMARK: Symphysis pubis

IMMOBILIZATION: Place hands on the chest or at patient's side. Prevent the body from touching the sides of the magnet by using sponges or sheets.

> **TIP:** The purpose of this study is to evaluate the extent of prostate disease and invasion. Primarily, we evaluate for spread from the central to peripheral zone and for invasion of seminal vesicles and neural bundles.

Acquisition of Axial Image of the Prostate

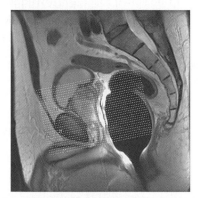

Figure 6-55 Sagittal image of the pelvis with axial locations for the prostate

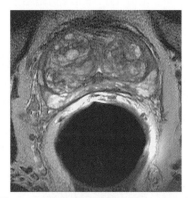

Figure 6-56 Axial image of the prostate

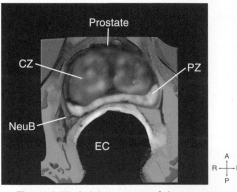

Figure 6-57 Axial anatomy of the prostate

KEY: CZ, central zone; **EC**, endorectal cell; **NeuB**, neural bundle; **PZ**, peripheral zone.

SLICE ACQUISITION: Superior to inferior
SLICE ALIGNMENT: Angle to the prostate
ANATOMIC COVERAGE: Superior to the seminal vesicles through the pubis

TIP: Ensure that the endo-rectal coil is positioned properly by evaluating the coil signal in the sagittal and coronal planes on the localizer.
   If the coil is not positioned properly, reposition it before continuing. Make sure the proper coil is selected before scanning.

Acquisition of Coronal Image of Prostate

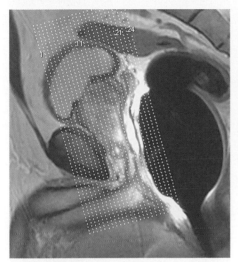

Figure 6-58 Sagittal image of the pelvis with coronal locations for the prostate

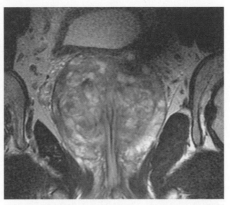

Figure 6-59 Coronal image of the prostate

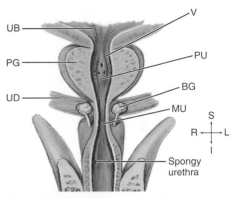

Figure 6-60 Coronal anatomy of the prostate

SLICE ACQUISITION: Anterior to posterior
SLICE ALIGNMENT: Align to prostate
ANATOMIC COVERAGE: Superior to seminal vesicles through the pubis

TIP: Make sure the proper coil is selected before scanning.

KEY: **BG**, bulbourethral gland; **MU**, membranous urethra; **PG**, prostate gland; **PU**, prostatic urethra; **UB**, urinary bladder; **UD**, urogenital diaphragm; **V**, verumontanum.

Acquisition of Sagittal Image

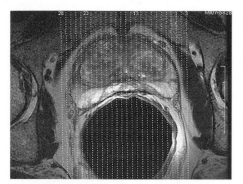

Figure 6-61 Axial image of the prostate with sagittal locations

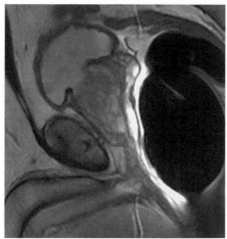

Figure 6-62 Sagittal image of the prostate

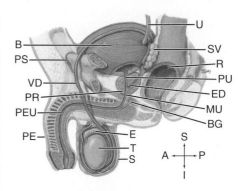

Figure 6-63 Sagittal anatomy of the prostate

SLICE ACQUISITION: Left to right
SLICE ALIGNMENT: Parallel to prostate
ANATOMIC COVERAGE: Superior seminal vesicles through the prostate

TIP: Make sure the proper coil is selected before scanning.

KEY: B, bladder; **BG,** bulbourethral gland; **E,** epididymis; **ED,** ejaculatory duct; **MU,** membranous urethra; **PE,** penis; **PEU,** penile urethra; **PR,** prostate; **PS,** public symphysis; **PU,** prostatic urethra; **R,** rectum; **S,** scrotum; **SV,** seminal vesicle; **T,** testis; **U,** ureter; **VD,** vas deferens.

Table 6-11 Male Pelvis: Prostate

Sequence 1.5	TR	TE	ETL or FA	Band-width	F Matrix	Ph Matrix	FOV	Slice Thick	Inter-space	NEX	TI	Pulse Sequence Options
Sag FRFSE	5000	102	20	41.67	320	224	24/.80	5.0	1.5	1		NPW
Ax T2 SSSFE	Min	90		62.50	384	224	40/.80	8.0	0	1		Asset, Sat S-I
Ax FRFSE	5000	102	20	41.67	320	224	18/18	4.0	0	2		Sat A-S, FC, NPW, Zip 512
Cor FRFSE	5000	102	20	41.67	320	224	18/18	4.0	.5	2		Sat A-S, FC, NPW, Zip 512
Sag FRFSE	5000	102	20	41.67	320	224	18/18	4.0	.5	4		Sat A-S, FC, NPW, Zip 512
Ax FGRE	350	In Ph	80	62.50	256	192	16/16	4.0	0	2		NPW, Zip 512

(Continued)

Table 6-11 Male Pelvis: Prostate—*cont'd*

Sequence 1.5	TR	TE	ETL or FA	Band-width	F Matrix	Ph Matrix	FOV	Slice Thick	Inter-space	NEX	TI	Pulse Sequence Options
Post GAD												
Ax Lava XV	Mach		12 FA	62.50	320	160	30/.90	4.4	0	1	66 loc/slab	Sat Special, Zip 2, Zip 512, Fluoro, Multiphase
Cor Lava XV	Mach		12 FA	62.50	320	192	32/.90	4.0	0	1	44 loc/slab	Sat Special, Zip 512

Sequence 3T	TR	TE	ETL or FA	Band-width	F Matrix	Ph Matrix	FOV	Slice Thick	Inter-space	NEX	TI	Pulse Sequence Options
Sag FRFSE	4000	102	20	41.67	320	192	24/.80	5.0	1.5	1		NPW
Ax T2 SSSFE	Min	90		62.50	384	224	40/.80	8.0	0	1		Asset, Sat S-I
Ax FRFSE	4200	140	24		62.50	320	224	14/14	3.0	0	2	Sat A-S, FC, NPW

Table 6-11	Male Pelvis: Prostate—*cont'd*												

Sequence 3T	TR	TE	ETL or FA	Band-width	F Matrix	Ph Matrix	FOV	Slice Thick	Inter-space	NEX	TI	Pulse Sequence Options
Cor FSE	4000	140	24	62.50	320	224	16/16	3.0	0	2		Sat A-S, FC, NPW
Sag FSE	4000	140	24	62.50	320	224	16/16	3.0	0	2		Sat A-S, FC, NPW, Zip 512
Ax GRE	300	In Ph	80	62.50	256	192	16/16	4.0	0	2		Fast, NPW, Zip 512
Post GAD												
Ax Lava	Mach		12 FA	83.33	320	192	30/.90	4.4	0	1	66 loc/ slab	Sat Special, Zip 2, Zip 512, Fluoro, Multiphase
Cor Lava	Mach		12 FA	83.33	320	192	32/.90	4.0	0	1	44 loc/ slab	Sat Special, Zip 2, Zip 512

Adjust FOV and loc/slab depending on patient's size.

Ax T2 SSFSE from the kidneys to the pubis.

Use a dielectric pad on the pelvis to suppress shading artifacts.

TRF (Tailor Radio-Frequency) should be used with all FSE sequence to increase # of slices per TR.

Perform LAVA sequence when contrast is ordered.

Table 6-12 Site Protocol: Male Pelvis: Prostate

Sequence 1.5	TR	TE	ETL or FA	Band-width	F Matrix	Ph Matrix	FOV	Slice Thick	Inter-space	NEX	TI	Pulse Sequence Options
Post GAD												

Sequence 3T	TR	TE	ETL or FA	Band-width	F Matrix	Ph Matrix	FOV	Slice Thick	Inter-space	NEX	TI	Pulse Sequence Options
Post GAD												

Table 6-12 Site Protocol: Male Pelvis: Prostate—*cont'd*

MRA OF THE RENAL ARTERIES

Acquire three-plane pilot of the abdomen per site specifications. Refer to images 6-1 through 6-3.

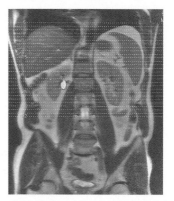

Figure 6-64 Coronal image of the abdomen with locs for acquisition of axial FIESTA

Figure 6-65 Axial image of the renal arteries

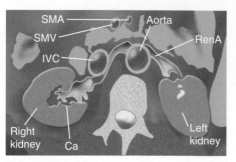

Figure 6-66 Axial anatomy of the renal arteries

KEY: **Ca**, calyx; **IVC**, inferior vena cava; **RenA**, renal artery; **SMA**, superior mesentric artery; **SMV**, superior mesentric vein.

TIP: Use manufacturer-specific fluoroscopic trigger to ensure proper visualization of contrast.

Have the patient go to the bathroom before positioning him or her on the table.

COIL: Multi-channel torso array or multi-channel cardiac coil

POSITION: Position the patient supine, feet first with the coil covering the diaphragm to the iliac crest.

LANDMARK: Midcoil

IMMOBILIZATION: Place the patient's arms over his or her head or elevated on cushions away from body.

Prevent the body from touching the sides of the magnet by using sponges or sheets.

Acquisition of Coronal FIESTA for the Renal Arteries

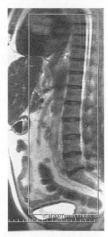

Figure 6-67 Sagittal image of the abdomen with locations for the acquisition of coronal FIESTA

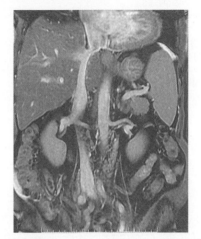

Figure 6-68 Coronal image of the renal arteries

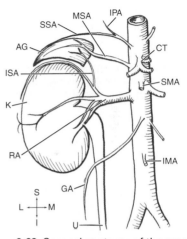

Figure 6-69 Coronal anatomy of the renal arteries

> ***KEY:*** **AG**, adrenal gland; **CT**, celiac trunk; **GA**, gonadal artery; **IMA**, inferior mesenteric artery; **IPA**, inferior phrenic artery; **ISA**, inferior suprarenal artery; **K**, kidney; **MSA**, middle suprarenal artery; **RA**, renal artery; **SMA**, superior mesenteric artery; **SSA**, superior suprarenal artery; **U**, ureter.

> ***TIP:*** Have the patient go to the bathroom before positioning.

COIL: Multi-channel torso array or multi-channel cardiac coil

POSITION: Supine, feet first, with coil covering xiphoid process to symphysis pubis. Place a cushion under the patient's knees.

LANDMARK: 2 inches above crest

IMMOBILIZATION: Place the hands above the patient's head or on the chest; hands may be secured with Velcro straps. Prevent the body from touching the sides of the magnet by using sponges or sheets.

Acquisition of 3D MRA Coronal Images of the Renal Arteries

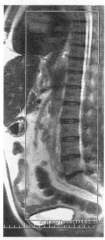

Figure 6-70 Sagittal image of the abdomen with coronal locations for the renal arteries

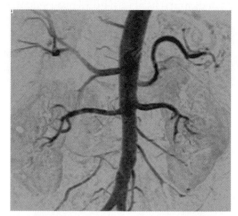

Figure 6-71 Coronal image of the renal arteries

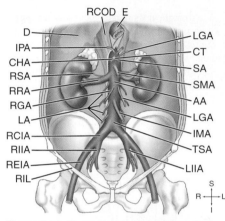

Figure 6-72 Coronal anatomy of the renal arteries

SLICE ACQUISITION: Anterior to posterior
SLICE ALIGNMENT: Straight, no angulation
ANATOMIC COVERAGE: T10 to L5 to include aortic-iliac bifurcation

TIP: Give the patient 5 seconds to hold his or her breath before the contrast acquisition. Use delayed K-space filling when available.

KEY: **AA**, abdominal aorta; **CHA**, common hepatic artery; **CT**, celiac trunk; **D**, diaphragm; **E**, esophagus; **IMA**, inferior mesenteric artery; **IPA**, inferior phrenic artery; **LA**, lumbar arteries; **LGA**, left gastric artery; **LGA**, left gonadal artery; **LIIA**, left internal iliac artery; **RCIA**, right common iliac artery; **RCOD**, right crus of diaphragm; **REIA**, right external iliac artery; **RGA**, right gonadal artery; **RIIA**, right internal iliac artery; **RIL**, right inguinal ligament; **RRA**, right renal artery; **RSA**, right suprarenal artery; **SA**, splenic artery; **SMA**, superior mesentric artery; **TSA**, terminal segment of the aorta.

Acquisition of Axial Phase Contrast Image of Renal Arteries

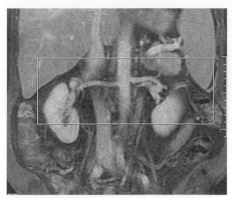

Figure 6-73 Coronal image of the abdomen with loc for axial PC of the renal arteries

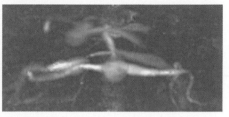

Figure 6-74 Axial image of the renal arteries

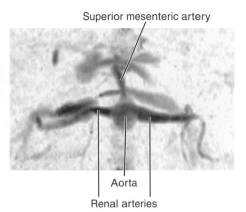

Figure 6-75 Axial anatomy of the renal arteries

SLICE ACQUISITION: Superior to inferior

SLICE ALIGNMENT: Straight, no angulation

ANATOMIC COVERAGE: Superior to inferior to the renal arteries

TIP: Use the reconstructed contrast-enhanced MRA coronal image for best visualization of both renal arteries.

Table 6-13 Renal Arteries

Sequence 1.5	TR	TE	ETL or FA	Band-width	F Matrix	Ph Matrix	FOV	Slice Thick	Inter-space	NEX	TI	Pulse Sequence Options
Cor T2 SSSFE	Min	90		62.50	384	224	48/.90	5	0	1		Asset, Sat S-I
Cor Fiesta	Min		70 FA	83.33	192	320	35/35	4	.4	1		Fast, Seq
Ax Fiesta	Min		70 FA	83.33	224	320	38/.80	4	.4	1		Fast, Seq, Sat Fat/Special
Ax T2 SSSFE	Min	90		62.50	384	224	40/.80	8	0	1		Asset, Sat S-I
Post GAD												
Cor 3D MRA C-+	Mach	Min	30 FA	50	320	192	36/.90	2.4	0	1	32 loc/ slab	Vas SPGR TOF, Fast, Zip 2, Zip 512, Fluoro Trigger, Multiphase

Table 6-13 Renal Arteries—*cont'd*

Sequence 1.5	TR	TE	ETL or FA	Band-width	F Matrix	Ph Matrix	FOV	Slice Thick	Inter-space	NEX	TI	Pulse Sequence Options
Ax 3D PC	25		45 FA	31.25	256	192	32/32	3	0	1	28 loc/slab	Vasc PC, FC, Vascular, Venc 40, Complex Diff, Direction all
Ax FSPGR	200	Min	90 FA	41.67	320	224	35	8	5	1		Sat F, FC

Sequence 3T	TR	TE	ETL or FA	Band-width	F Matrix	Ph Matrix	FOV	Slice Thick	Inter-space	NEX	TI	Pulse Sequence Options
Cor T2 SSSFE	Min	140		83.33	384	224	48/.90	7	0	1		Asset, Sat S-I
Cor Fiesta	Min		45 FA	125	160	160	35/35	4	.4	1		Fast, Seq
Ax Fiesta	Min		45 FA	83.33	192	160	38/.80	4	.4	1		Fast, Seq, Sat Fat/Special

(Continued)

Table 6-13 Renal Arteries—*cont'd*

Sequence 3T	TR	TE	ETL or FA	Band-width	F Matrix	Ph Matrix	FOV	Slice Thick	Inter-space	NEX	TI	Pulse Sequence Options
Ax T2 SSSFE	Min	100		83.33	288	192	40/.80	8	0	1		Asset, Sat S-I
Post GAD												
Cor 3D MRA C-+	Mach	Min	30 FA	62.50	320	192	36/.90	2.4	0	.75	32 loc/slab	Vas SPGR TOF, Fast, Zip 2, Zip 512, Fluoro Trigger, Multiphase
Ax 3D PC	22		25 FA	31.25	256	192	32/32	3	0	1	28 loc/slab	Vasc PC, FC, Vascular, Venc 40, Complex Diff, Direction all
Ax FSPGR	200	Min	90 FA	62.50	320	224	35	8	5	1		Sat F, FC

FOV and loc/slab are dependent on patient's size.
Make sure to keep the breath-hold sequences approximately 20 seconds.
The coronal 3D MRA is a dynamic three phases per location, 1 pre-GAD and 2 post-GAD. Auto subtraction is used for best contrast enhancement.
Use a 5-second scan delay after each phase.
A non–contrast-enhanced MRA should be performed when available.

| Table 6-14 | Site Protocol: Renal Arteries |

Sequence 1.5	TR	TE	ETL or FA	Band-width	F Matrix	Ph Matrix	FOV	Slice Thick	Inter-space	NEX	TI	Pulse Sequence Options
Post GAD												

(Continued)

Table 6-14 Site Protocol: Renal Arteries—*cont'd*

Sequence 3T	TR	TE	ETL or FA	Band-width	F Matrix	Ph Matrix	FOV	Slice Thick	Inter-space	NEX	TI	Pulse Sequence Options
Post GAD												

MRA RUNOFF—ABDOMEN, PELVIS, AND LOWER EXTREMITIES

Acquire Fast TOF locations for the top, middle, and lower extremities; reference images below.

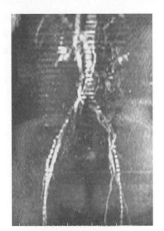

Figure 6-76

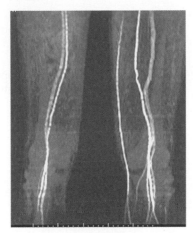

Figure 6-77

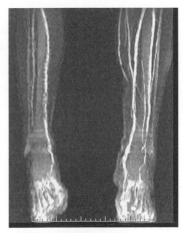

Figure 6-78

COIL: Peripheral vascular or CTL, or multi-channel torso
POSITION: Supine, feet first, legs flat
LANDMARK: When using PV coil with three stations, landmark the mid top station.
When using CTL coil, landmark the mid lower leg.
IMMOBILIZATION: Place arms at sides, and support with table straps.
Prevent the body from touching the sides of the magnet by using sponges or sheets.

TIP: Place MR-compatible blood pressure cuffs on thighs to delay venous flow enhancement to the lower extremities.
Inflate the cuffs after the mask and before contrast injection.

Acquisition of Upper Runoff Images—Aortal Through Femoral Vessels

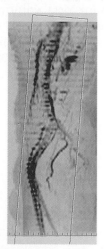

Figure 6-79 Sagittal rotation of the upper TOF image with coronal locations

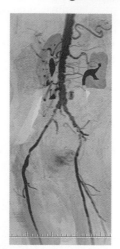

Figure 6-80 Coronal image of the abdominal vessels

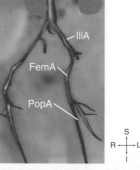

Figure 6-81 Coronal anatomy of the abdominal vessels

KEY: **AbAor**, abdominal aorta; **FemA**, femoral artery; **ILiA**, iliac artery; **PopA**, popliteal artery.

SLICE ACQUISITION: Anterior to posterior

SLICE ALIGNMENT: Parallel to aorta and iliac branches

ANATOMIC COVERAGE: From superior mesenteric artery to proximal iliac arteries, overlap the top and middle sections by at least 4 cm.

TIP: Masks are acquired first followed by contrast acquisition. When rotating the images into the sagittal plane, ensure superimposition of the vessels.

Acquisition of Middle Runoff Images—Femoral Through Popliteal Vessels

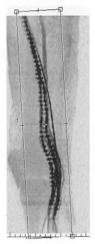

Figure 6-82 Sagittal rotation of the middle TOF image with coronal locations

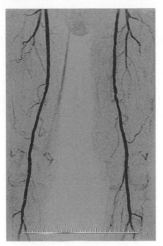

Figure 6-83 Coronal image of the femoral vessels

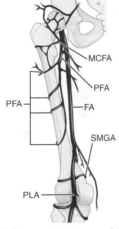

Figure 6-84 Coronal anatomy of the femoral vessels

KEY: **FA**, femoral artery; **MCFA**, medial circumflex femoral artery; **PFA**, perforating arteries; **PFA**, profunda femoris artery; **PLA**, popliteal artery; **SMGA**, superior medial genicular artery.

SLICE ACQUISITION: Anterior to posterior

SLICE ALIGNMENT: Parallel to the femoral arteries

ANATOMIC COVERAGE: From above the ischium through the knee joint, overlapping the upper and lower stations by at least 4 cm

TIP: All three acquisitions (upper, middle, and lower) are acquired simultaneously. Masks are acquired first, followed by contrast acquisition. When rotating the images into the sagittal plane, ensure superimposition of the vessels.

Acquisition of Lower Runoff Images—Popliteal Through Plantar Vessels

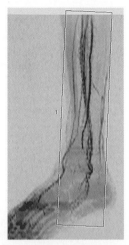

Figure 6-85 Sagittal rotation of the lower TOF image with coronal locations

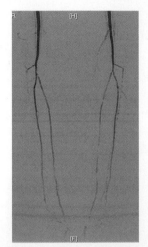

Figure 6-86 Coronal image of the vessels in the lower leg and foot

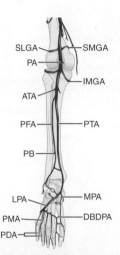

Figure 6-87 Coronal anatomy of the vessels in the lower leg and foot

SLICE ACQUISITION: Anterior to posterior

SLICE ALIGNMENT: Parallel to the vessels of the lower leg

ANATOMIC COVERAGE: From the tibial plateau to the phalanges of the foot, overlapping the middle and lower station by at least 4 cm

TIP: Masks are acquired first, followed by contrast acquisition. When rotating the images into the sagittal plane, ensure superimposition of the vessels.

KEY: **ATA**, anterior tibial artery; **DBDPA**, deep branch of dorsalis pedis artery; **IMGA**, inferior medial genicular artery; **LPA**, lateral plantar artery; **MPA**, medial plantar artery; **PA**, popliteal artery; **PB**, perforating branch; **PDA**, plantar digital arteries; **PFA**, peroneal (fibular) artery; **PMA**, plantar metatarsal artery; **PTA**, posterior tibial artery; **SLGA**, superior lateral genicular artery; **SMGA**, superior medial genicular artery.

Runoff Images

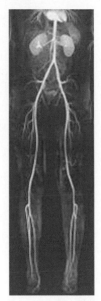

Figure 6-88 Three-section MRA runoff

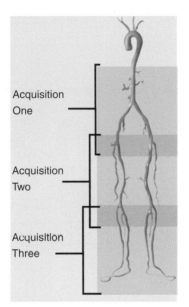

Figure 6-89 Structural references demonstrating overlap

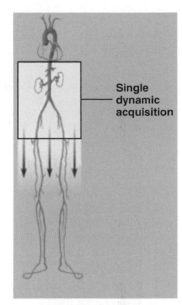

Figure 6-90 MRA runoff

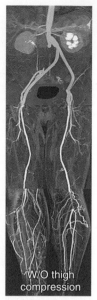

Figure 6-91 MRA runoff without thigh cuffs

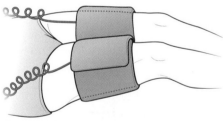

Figure 6-92 Proper positioning of thigh cuffs

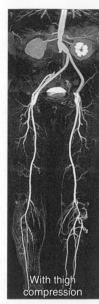

Figure 6-93 MRA runoff using thigh cuffs

Table 6-15 Runoff MRA of the Abdomen and Lower Extremities

Sequence 1.5	TR	TE	ETL or FA	Band-width	F Matrix	Ph Matrix	FOV	Slice Thick	Inter-space	NEX	TI	Pulse Sequence Options
Fast TOF Loc	Min	Min	60 FA	31.25	256	128	48/.75	5	0	1		Vasc TOF SPGR, Fast, FC, Sat Gap 10, seq
Post GAD												
Cor Tricks LL	4.5	Min	45 FA	62.50	512	224	48/.90	3	0	1		Zip 2, Pause On, Temporal Resolution of 7-10 depending on patient pathology, 15 phases
3D Top MRA	Mach	Min	30 FA	83.33	512	192	48/.80	3.6	0	.75	36 Loc/slab	Vasc TOF SPGR, Fast, Multistation, Fluoro, Zip 4, Zip 512
3D Mid MRA	Mach	Min	30 FA	83.33	384	192	48/.80	3.6	0	.75	36 Loc/slab	Vasc TOF SPGR, Fast, Multistation, Zip 4, Zip 512
3D Lower MRA	Mach	Min	30 FA	62.50	512	384	46/.70	2.4	0	.75	36 Loc/slab	Vasc TOF SPGR, Fast, Multistation, Zip 4, Zip 512

(Continued)

Table 6-15 Runoff MRA of the Abdomen and Lower Extremities—*cont'd*

Sequence 3T	TR	TE	ETL or FA	Band-width	F Matrix	Ph Matrix	FOV	Slice Thick	Inter-space	NEX	TI	Pulse Sequence Options
Fast TOF Loc	Min	Min	90 FA	31.25	256	128	48/.75	5	0	1		Vasc TOF SPGR, Fast, FC, Sat Gap 10, Seq
Post GAD												
Cor Tricks LL	3.5	Min	35 FA	62.50	384	320	46/.90	3	0	.75		Zip 2, Pause On, Temporal Resolution of 7-10 depending on patient pathology, 15 phases
3D Top MRA	Mach	Min	30 FA	83.33	320	192	46/.80	3.6	0	.75	36 Loc/ slab	Vasc TOF SPGR, Fast, Multistation, Fluoro, Zip 4, Zip 512
3D Mid MRA	Mach	Min	30 FA	83.33	320	192	46/.80	3.6	0	.75	36 Loc/ slab	Vasc TOF SPGR, Fast, Multistation, Zip 4, Zip 512
3D Lower MRA	Mach	Min	30 F	83.33	512	384	46/.70	2.4	0	.75	36 Loc/ slab	Vasc TOF SPGR, Fast, Multistation, Zip 4, Zip 512

Repeat fast TOF loc three times for the top, middle and bottom localization.
These locs can be used to prescribe the runoff top, middle and lower levels.
Choose a PV coil which has a top, mid and lower coil, each which corresponds to the abdomen, pelvis and lower extremities.
CTL coil top, mid and lower and torso coils can also be used.

Table 6-16 Site Protocol: Runoff MRA of the Abdomen and Lower Extremities

Sequence 1.5	TR	TE	ETL or FA	Band-width	F Matrix	Ph Matrix	FOV	Slice Thick	Inter-space	NEX	TI	Pulse Sequence Options
Post GAD												

Sequence 3T	TR	TE	ETL or FA	Band-width	F Matrix	Ph Matrix	FOV	Slice Thick	Inter-space	NEX	TI	Pulse Sequence Options
Post GAD												

APPENDIX A

Gadolinium-Based Contrast Agents (GBCAs)

Gadolinium-Containing Contrast Agents (GBCAs) are used to improve visualization of tumors, abscesses, inflammation, blood vessels and other anatomic structures in MRI and MRA. Gadolinium is a paramagnetic MRI contrast agent which shortens the T1 and T2 relaxation time of protons.

T1 images are normally acquired to demonstrate anatomic structures while T2 images are normally acquired to demonstrate pathology associated with fluid, tumor or infection. Lesions on MR can be missed since both water and tumors can exhibit low T1 signal intensity.

In order to increase contrast signal between pathology and normal tissue extracellular gadolinium based contrast agents (GBCA) were developed. The primary effect of these agents is shortening the T1 relaxation time which affects image contrast on T1-weighted images. Reduction of T1 relaxation time results in bright signal and increased intensity of any lesion that takes up the GBCA.

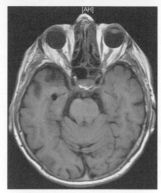

T1 axial brain pre-GAD

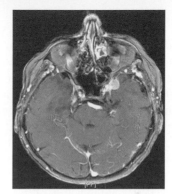

T1 axial brain post-GAD

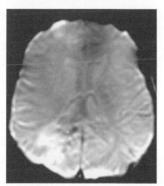

T2* (perfusion) axial brain pre-GAD

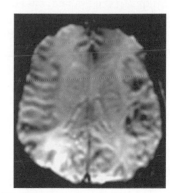

T2* (perfusion) axial brain post-GAD

GBCA can also shorten T2 relaxation times causing both T2 and T2* signals to be reduced. Since bright lesions are easier to see than dark lesions, GBCA are primarily used with T1-weighted images where enhancing lesions will be bright.

GBCA is a paramagnetic substance that has seven unpaired electrons in the outer orbit affecting the local magnetic field near the gadolinium atom. As water protons pass by the gadolinium, a "moderate positive effect" from these gadolinium induced fluctuations occurs in the local magnetic field, near the Larmor frequency. This effect shortens the T1 relaxation time. In its free state, gadolinium is a heavy metal that is toxic if it remains in the body for a long period of time. As a contrast agent gadolinium is tightly bound to a chelate to prevent heavy metal toxicity and to ensure excretion from the body by the kidneys.

Gadolinium will not cross the intact blood-brain barrier unless there is a disruption. Therefore, gadolinium does not enhance normal brain or lesions that have a normal blood-brain barrier. However, disruption of the blood-brain barrier and abnormal vascularity allows enhancement of lesions including neoplasms, abscesses, and infarcts since the gadolinium leaks into the abnormal or damaged tissue in and around these lesions. Gadolinium enhances highly vascular normal structures of the brain including the pituitary gland, choroid plexus, transverse sinuses, and veins and arteries. Gadolinium enhances the vascular structures and distributes into the interstitial space and is eliminated from the body primarily through the kidneys.

After gadolinium administration, T1 weighted spin echo or spoiled gradient echo scans are performed and pathology and vascular structures of the body will enhance. T2* scans (example brain perfusion) are performed to exploit the agents' magnetic susceptibility and T2 shortening effects, causing vascular signal to reduce (see p. 349).

The use of gadolinium in MR imaging is used routinely for brain, spine for disk vs. scar, metastatic lesion, MS activity, infection, body imaging, dynamic liver, breast and cardiac imaging. Dynamic imaging has the ability to look at the kinetics of lesion enhancement. MRA with gadolinium is routinely performed for the chest, abdomen, pelvis, lower extremity run-offs, vascular structures of the head and neck. Gadolinium is also injected intra-articularly in orthopedic imaging for MR arthrography.

Gadolinium is not approved for all body applications although radiologists commonly use contrast media for a clinical purpose not contained in the labeling which is known as "off-label" use. By definition, such usage is not specifically approved by the Food and Drug Administration and companies are not legally entitled to market GBCA for "off label" indications. However, the FDA does not regulate the practice of medicine by physicians and states that physicians have some latitude in using gadolinium chelates off label as guided by clinical circumstances and the published literature. Radiologists should be prepared to justify such usage in individual cases. Examples include MR angiography, cardiac and abdominal applications, and pediatric applications in patients younger than two years of age. It is suggested that the package insert be reviewed whenever decisions are made to use contrast.

GBCA can be classified as cyclic or linear compounds depending whether or not the chelate completely encircles the gadolinium with strong covalent bonds. Another classification is ionic or nonionic similar to the classification of iodinated contrast. It is noted that cyclic and ionic gadolinium compounds are considered less likely to release the gadolinium ion and hence the most safe, from the point of view of Gadolinium toxicity. The FDA approved GBCA include Omniscan, Multihance, Magnevist, ProHance and OptiMARK .

Eovist and Ablavar are newly FDA approved contrast with very specific indications. Eovist (Gadoxetate Disodium) is the first organ specific MRI contrast to detect and characterize malignant and benign focal liver lesions. ABLAVAR (Gadofosveset Trisodium) is a FDA blood pool contrast agent approved for MRA to evaluate aortoiliac occlusive disease in patients with known or suspected peripheral vascular disease.

- Magnevist (gadopentetate dimeglumine), Eovist, Ablavar and MultiHance (gadobenate dimeglumine) have the linear structure and are ionic.
- Omniscan (gadodiamide) and OptiMARK (gadoversetamide) have the linear structure and are nonionic.
- ProHance (gadoteridol) has a cyclic structure and is nonionic.

ProHance is considered to have the highest thermodynamic and conditional stability, and Omniscan/Optimark the weakest. All the above GBCA are solely excreted by the kidneys except Eovist, Ablavar and MultiHance which have two unique properties; elimination through both the kidneys and liver and higher T1 relaxivity. These features are advantageous for imaging of the CNS, liver and for MRA. Eovist has the highest liver excretion which is approximately 50 percent eliminated through the liver and 50 percent eliminated through the kidney while Multihance has a 4% liver/biliary excretion.

Oral contrasts such as VoLumen are sorbital solutions with a small amount of barium suspension which distends the bowel. Sorbital is a sugar which the body does not absorb and remains in the intestinal lumen creating an osmotic pressure that distends the bowel. It can be advantageous for pelvic imaging, particularly for diseases of the colon such as colon cancer,

Crohns and other inflammatory diseases, as well as possible appendicitis in pregnant women. Natural products with high manganese concentration such as blueberries, pineapple juice and green tea can also be used for T1 contrast enhancement effect.

MRI contrast has always been considered to be extremely safe and has been used "off label" at double and triple doses particularly for MRA studies. In May 2007, the FDA notified healthcare professionals of the "black boxed warning" about the risk of NSF (Nephrogenic Systemic Fibrosis). The risk for NSF/NSD (Nephrogenic Fibrosing Dermopathy) presents in patients with acute or chronic renal insufficiency and patients with renal dysfunction due to the hepatorenal syndrome, or in the perioperative liver transplantation period. Patients who develop NSF/NSD have areas of hardening and tightening of the skin with joint stiffness and muscle weakness as well as scarring of their body organs. Patients who developed NSF were either on dialysis or had severe renal inefficiency and were given high-doses of gadolinium.

Patients with acute or chronic severe renal insufficiency (GFR, glomerular filtration rate < 30mL/min/1.73m2), hepatorenal syndrome, or in the perioperative liver transplantation period should avoid use of GBCA unless the diagnostic information is essential. All patients with renal dysfunction should be screened by obtaining a history and/or serum creatinine.

When administering a GBCA:
- Do not exceed the FDA recommended dose stated in product insert.
- Allow sufficient time for the elimination of the GBCA prior to any re-administration. Twenty-four hours is recommended.
- All dosing should be calculated by weight (kg).
- Screening patients for renal disease based on history is sufficient. Patients with no history of renal disease (stated or documented) do not need laboratory studies prior to administration.
- Patients with a positive history of renal disease must have a recent serum creatinine.
- Review the most recent ACR Manual of Contrast Media Version 7, 2010 for details.
- The estimated GFR (glomerular filtration rate) can be calculated using the MDRD method with inputs of serum creatinine, age, gender and race. The MDRD method can be found at: http://nephron.com/cgi-bin/MDRD_NKF.cgi. This calculator is calibrated for adults age 18 to 70.
- As stated in the recent ACR Guidelines (7 Contrast media in children, pg 4) There is no perfect manner of estimating the GFR in children. The National Kidney Disease Education Program (NKDEP) (an initiative of the National Institutes of Health (NIH)) has published the following informa-

tion regarding the estimation of GFR in children. A pediatric calculation is also available at http://nkdep.nih.gov/professionals/gfr_calculators/gfr_children.htm

- GBCA should be avoided in patients with severe renal insufficiency or renal failure unless the diagnostic information is essential and not available with non-contrast enhanced magnetic resonance imaging (MRI). This is especially true for patients not on hemodialysis.
- Patients on hemodialysis can receive contrast but should have hemodialysis scheduled the same day following the exam and no more than 24 hours after receiving contrast.

FDA BLACK BOX WARNING on all GBMCA

Warning: Nephrogenic Systemic Fibrosis

Gadolinium-based contrast agents increase the risk for nephrogenic systemic fibrosis (NSF) in patients with:

- acute or chronic severe renal insufficiency (glomerular filtration rate <30mL/min/1.73m^2), or
- acute renal insufficiency of any severity due to the hepato-renal syndrome or in the perioperative liver transplantation period.

In these patients, avoid use of gadolinium-based contrast agents unless the diagnostic information is essential and not available with non-contrast enhanced magnetic resonance imaging (MRI). NSF may result in fatal or debilitating systemic fibrosis affecting the skin, muscle and internal organs. Screen all patients for renal dysfunction by obtaining a history and/or laboratory tests. When administering a gadolinium-based contrast agent, do not exceed the recommended dose and allow a sufficient period of time for elimination of the agent from the body prior to any readministration

(See WARNINGS).

The U.S. Food and Drug Administration have asked manufacturers to include the above **"Black Box Warning"** on all gadolinium-based magnetic resonance contrast agents. They also issued a "Dear Healthcare Professional" letter dated September 12, 2007 to notify all Radiologists, Nephrologists, Dermatologists and other healthcare professionals of the addition **"Black Box Warning."**

ADVERSE EVENTS

The most common reactions are 9.8% headaches, 4.1% nausea, and 2% vomiting, less than 1% hypotensive gastro-intestinal upset, rash and deaths have been reported.

Adverse Event	Multihance Gadobenate dimeglumine (N=2367)	Magnevist Gadopentetate dimeglumine (N=1068)	ProHance Gadoteridol (N=1709)	Omniscan Gadodiamide (N=700)	OptiMARK Gadoversetamide (N=1663)
Headache (%)	1.9	3.6	0.4	4.4	7.5
Nausea (%)	1.3	1.5	1.1	3.6	2.6
Taste perversion (%)	1.1	0.3	1.2	2.1	5.7
Urticaria (%)	0.3	0.3	0.4	0.1	N/A

From Molecule to Magnet: A Literature Review of Gadobenate Dimeglumine.

Anaphylactic reactions have been reported and in many of these instances the patient had a history of respiratory difficulty or an allergic respiratory problem, such as asthma. Package inserts have warnings regarding patients with known allergic respiratory disease.

The exact incidence of severe anaphylactic reactions is unknown but appears to be between 1:100,000 to 1:500,000. As with iodinated contrast, there is evidence that nonionic GBCA have a lower incidence of adverse events compared to ionic GBCA. Approximately 80% of gadolinium is excreted by the kidneys in three hours. There are also agents that are partially excreted through the liver. About 98% is recovered by feces and urine in one week. Package inserts should be considered in all cases.

The ACR guidelines "Contrast Agent Safety" regarding adverse events should always be followed. It states that patients with asthma and history of allergic respiratory disorders are at a higher risk of adverse events. Previous adverse events to iodinated or

MRI contrast should also be considered a higher risk of adverse event since they are more than twice as likely to have a reaction to gadolinium. Patients who have previously reacted to one MR contrast agent can be injected with another agent if they are restudied. Pre-medication with corticosteroids and occasionally antihistamines is prudent.

Since patients receiving MR contrast agents have the potential for adverse event, it is prudent to have appropriate monitoring equipment and accessories readily available for the proper management and support for the patients. Routinely monitoring the patient's electrocardiogram (ECG) and oxygen saturation is crucial. A MR compatible physiologic monitoring system should be used to avoid burns, projectiles or other MR related issues. Most systems have the ability to monitor the heart and respiratory rate, blood pressure, and oxygen saturation.

PREGNANCY

MR contrast crosses the placental barrier and appears within the fetal bladder only moments after intravenous administration. Since the clearance rate of gadolinium contrast agents from the amniotic fluid is unknown the administration to pregnant patients is not recommended unless the benefit out ways risk to the fetus. A written informed consent should be obtained prior to administration.

BREAST FEEDING MOTHERS

Since MR contrast is excreted in very low concentrations in human breast milk over approximately 33 hours, it is recommended that nursing mothers do not breastfeed for 36 to 48 hours after administration. When scheduling the patient who is breast feeding it is recommended to inform them to pump breast milk prior to the study, if necessary.

PEDIATRIC PATIENTS

For pediatric patients the only contrast that is approved for children over 2 years of age is Magnevist, Multihance and Prohance. None of the contrast agents are approved for children less than 2 years of age, since the safety of these agents has not been established. However, there have been no adverse clinical events reported in association with the use of MR imaging contrast agents in this pediatric group.

CONTRAST WRITTEN ORDERS AND ADMINISTRATION:

- Since MR contrast agents are considered a medication, standard medical practice should include a written and signed order from a radiologist and or physician.

- The order must include the patient's name, date, specified brand GBCA, dose, route and rate of administration.
- The approved FDA dosage per kg of weight, for a particular agent, should be administrated.
- The ACR approves of the injection of contrast agent by certified and/or licensed radiologic technologists and radiologic nurses under the direction of a radiologist or physician's designee who is personally and immediately available.

CONTRAST AND NSF/NSD:

Some renal insufficient patients who received "higher than standard dose" of GBCA developed NSF, which is an incurable skin disease that hardens the skin from the outside/in. As stated earlier in 2006-2007 the FDA issued a black box warning for GBCA. Gadolinium in its original state is toxic and need chelates to remove it from the body. One theory regarding issues with impaired renal patients is that since they are on many medications, including potassium, zinc, iron and calcium, the chelate of the gadolinium ion is pulled or dissociated from the gadolinium by the other medications. This dissociation occurs by a process known as transmetallation, whereby other cations replace the gadolinium associated with the chelate. When this happens free gadolinium remaining in the body and is sometimes trapped by binding to phosphates which are elevated in patients in renal failure and on dialysis. Without normal renal function the gadolinium cannot be cleared from the body and stays around possibly causing this debilitating disease. This is only a theory and not proven. What is proven and documented in the ACR Guidance Document for Safe MR Practices 2007 and by the FDA, is that the least stable contrast agents were implicated as a higher risk in more of the documented cases.

In the recent ACR Manual of Contrast Media Version 7, 2010, contrast media has been catorgized in three groups as follows. It is recommend that all read the Contrast Manual in its entirety.

Group I: Agents associated with the greatest number of NSF cases:

Gadodiamide (Omniscan® – GE Healthcare)

Gadopentetate dimeglumine (Magnevist® – Bayer HealthCare Pharmaceuticals) Gadoversetamide (OptiMARK® – Covidien)

Group II: Agents associated with few, if any, unconfounded cases of NSF:

Gadobenate dimeglumine (MultiHance® – Bracco Diagnostics)

Gadoteridol (ProHance® – Bracco Diagnostics)

Gadoteric acid (Dotarem® – Guerbet) - as of this writing not FDA-approved for use in the United States.

Gadobutrol (Gadovist® – Bayer HealthCare Pharmaceuticals) – as of this writing not FDA-approved for use in the United States.

Group III: Agents which have only recently appeared on the market in the US:

Gadofosveset (Ablavar® – Lantheus Medical Imaging)

Gadoxetic acid (Eovist® – Bayer HealthCare Pharmaceuticals)

On September 9, 2010, the U.S. Food and Drug Administration (FDA) announced that it is requiring that GBCAs carry new warnings on their labels about the risk of a rare and potentially fatal condition known as "nephrogenic systemic fibrosis (NSF)," if the drug is administered to certain patients with kidney disease.

Three of the GBCAs—Magnevist, Omniscan, and Optimark—will be described as inappropriate for use among patients with acute kidney injury or chronic severe kidney disease. All GBCA labels will emphasize the need to screen patients to detect these types of kidney dysfunctions before administration.

LEGAL RAMIFICATIONS OF CONTRAST

Hundreds of lawsuits have been initiated and numerous legal websites have published the NSF-MRI implication with comments like:

- "Have you had MRI Dye?"
- "If you or a loved one has experienced a skin disorder called Nephrogenic Systemic Fibrosis (NSF, also known as Nephrogenic Fibrosing Dermopathy, NFD) – sustained as a result of the injection of a gadolinium based contrast agent used in MRIs and MRAs (gadodiamide), you may have a lawsuit that should be pursued".
- "MRI Contrast Dye Could Cause Incurable Disease, Gadolinium Blamed For the Problems"
- "Contrast Dye Responsible For Serious Side Effects"
- "Injured by Gadolinium?"

During our research we found hundreds of advertisements from legal websites with regard to MRI contrast. Practices have received many questions from patients and patient's families who had scans in 2006 and 2007 particularly wanting to know "what brand of contrast" they received at the time of their MRI scan. These become Risk Management issues and should never be handled by the MRI technologist.

It is important to note that the MRI industry has completely changed practices when it comes to the administration of contrast and all should remember to strictly follow the ACR and FDA guidelines. MRI Institutional Contrast Policies are recommended and should be reviewed often by a team of physicians, nurses and technologists making sure all understand what has been written and agreed to. All MR departments should have a "MRI safety officer" who oversees all MRI policies including contrast.

Bibliography

American College of Radiology: *Manual on contrast media*, vol 7. Available at: http://www.acr.org/SecondaryMainMenuCategories/quality_safety/contrast_manual.aspx.

American College of Radiology: *Joint Commission Issues Sentinel Event Alert on MRI Safety*, Available at: http://www.acr.org/SecondaryMainMenuCategories/quality_safety/MRSafety/JointCommissionIssuesMRISentinelEventAlert.aspx.

American College of Radiology: *Manual on contrast media*, vol 7, Reston, VA, 2010, American College of Radiology.

American College of Radiology: *MR Safety*, Available at: http://www.acr.org/SecondaryMainMenuCategories/quality_safety/MRSafety.aspx.

Cerqueira MD, Weissman NJ, Dilsizian V, et al: Standardized myocardial segmentation and nomenclature for tomographic imaging of the heart: a statement for healthcare professionals from the Cardiac Imaging Committee of the Council on Clinical Cardiology of the American Heart Association, *Circulation* 105:539, 2002.

Coakley FV, Glenn OA, Qayyam A, et al: Fetal MRI: a developing technique for the developing patient, *AJR* 182:243–252, 2004.

Friedrich MG, et al: Cardiovascular magnetic resonance in myocarditis: a JACC white paper, *J Am Coll Cardiol* 53:1475–1487, 2009.

Haaga J, Lanzieri C, Gilkenson R: *CT and MRI imaging of the whole body*, St Louis, 2003, Mosby.

Huang L, Wong XH, Liu SR, et al: The application of DWI and ADC map in cerebral infarction, *Proc Intl Soc Mag Reson Med* 9:1446, 2001.

International Society for Magnetic Resonance in Medicine: *Gadolinium-Based Contrast Agents for Magnetic Resonance Imaging Scans (marketed as Omniscan, OptiMARK, Magnevist, ProHance, and MultiHance)*. Available at: www.ismrm.org/special/FDA%20gadolinium1206.pdf.

Kanel E: *Magnetic resonance safe practice guidelines of the University of Pittsburgh Medical Center*, 2001.

Kanel E, Barkovich AJ, Bell C, et al: *ACR guidance document for safe MRI practices*, 2007, ACR.org.

Kelly L, Peterson C: *Sectional anatomy for imaging professionals*, St Louis, 2007, Mosby.

McGee KP, Williamson EE, Julsrud P: *Mayo Clinic guide to cardiac magnetic resonance imaging*, ed 1, London, 2008, Informa Healthcare.

McRobbie D, et al: *MRI from picture to proton*, New York, 2003, Cambridge University Press.

Medicexchange.com: *FDA Approves Eovist® to Detect and Characterize Focal Liver Lesions*, Available at: http://www.medicexchange.com/Bayer-Healthcare/fda-approves-eovistr-to-detect-and-characterize-focal-liver-lesions.html.

Moeller T, Reif E: *MRI parameters and positioning*, Stuttgart, 2003, Thieme. MRI Safety.com.

Murphy KPJ, Szopinski KT, Cohan RH, et al: Occurrence of adverse reaction to gadolinium-based contrast material and management of patients at increased risk, *Acad Radiol* 6:656–664, 1999.

Prince M : Molecule to Magnet: A Literature Review of Gadobenate Dimeglumine.

Prince M, Grist T, Debatin J: *3D contrast MR angiography*, New York, 2003, Springer.

Reyes, Bartolomei, Brown: Gadolinium Dangers, Available at: http://www.reyeslaw.com/dangerous-drugs/gadolinium.asp.

Runge V: *Contrast enhanced clinical magnetic resonance imaging*, Lexington, 1997, University Press of Kentucky.

Schoenberg SO, Zech CJ, Panteleon A, et al: New perspectives and challenges in abdominal 3T MR imaging, *Appl Radiol* 36(suppl):2007. Available at:

http://www.appliedradiology.com/articles/Article.asp?ID=1330&IssueID=1 70&ThreadID= Accessed May 29, 2008.

Shellock F: *Reference manual for magnetic resonance safety implants and devices*, Los Angeles, 2009, Bracco.

Shellock R: *Magnetic resonance procedures; health effects and safety*, Boca Raton, FL, 2000, CRC Press.

The Joint Commission: *MRI Sentinel Events*, Available at: http://www.joint-commission.org/SentinelEvents/.

United States Food and Drug Administration: *Gadolinium-containing Contrast Agents for Magnetic Resonance Imaging (MRI): Magnevist, MultiHance, Omniscan, OptiMARK, ProHance*, Available at: http://www. fda.gov/Safety/MedWatch/SafetyInformation//ucm152672.htm.

United States Food and Drug Administration: *New warnings required for on use of gadolinium-based contrast agents*, Available at: http://www.fda.gov/ NewsEvents/Newsroom/PressAnnouncements/ucm225286.htm.

United States Food and Drug Administration: *FDA Drug Safety Communication: New warnings for using gadolinium-based contrast agents in patients with kidney dysfunction.* Available at: http://www.fda.gov/Drugs/ DrugSafety/ucm223966.htm.

United States Food and Drug Administration: *Important Drug Warning for Gadolinium-Based Contrast Agents.* Available at: http://imaging.bayer-healthcare.com/html/pdfs/magnevist/DDRletter.pdf.

Verma SK, Mitchell DG: *Liver metastasis on diffusion-weighted MRI.* Available at:http://www.dograrad.com/teaching-case/gi-radiology/20100202/liver-metastasis-diffusion-weighted-mri-422.html.

Contrast Agents References

Bracco: Multihance and ProHance
http://www.multihanceusa.com/home.htm
http://dailymed.nlm.nih.gov/dailymed/drugInfo.cfm?id=8929
Bayer: Magnevist, and Eovist
http://imaging.bayerhealthcare.com/html/magnevist/index.html
General Electric Medical: Omniscan
http://www.gehealthcare.com/caen/md/omniscan.html
Covidien: OptiMARK
http://imaging.covidien.com/covidienImaging/pageBuilder.aspx?topicID=132 292&page=Catalog:Model
Ezem: Volumen
http://www.ezem.com/pdf/1304080_ct.pdfhttp://www.ezem.com/ pdf/1304080_ct.pdf
Lantheus Medical Imaging: ABLAVAR
http://www.lantheus.com/News-Press-2009-1008.html

B

VENDOR MRI ACRONYMS

	Siemens	GE	Phillips	Toshiba
Patient Orientation Sequence	*Localizer, Scout*	*Localizer*	*Plan Scan*	*Localizer*
Sequence Type				
Spin Echo	SE	SE	SE	SE
Gradient Echo	GRE	GRE	Fast Field Echo (FFE)	Field Echo (FE)
Spoiled Gradient Echo	FLASH/T1 FISP	SPGR/MPSPGR	T1-FFE	RF spoiled/FE
Coherent Gradient Echo	FISP	GRASS	FFE	FFE
Balanced GE	True FISP	FIESTA	Balanced FFE	True SSFP
Multi-Echo Data Image Combination	MEDIC	MERGE	mFFE	FE 3D dual
Ultrafast Gradient Echo	Turbo FLASH	Fast GRE, Fast SPGR	TFE	Fast FE

(Continued)

	Siemens	GE	Phillips	Toshiba
Ultrafast Gradient Echo 3D	MPRAGE	3D FGRE, 3D Fast SPGR	3D TFE	3D Fast FE
Volume Interpolated GRE	VIBE	FAME, LAVA	THRIVE	VIBE
Susceptibility-Weighted Imaging	SWI	SWI/SWAN	Venous BOLD	FSBB-HOP
Dynamic/ Time Resolved Imaging	TWIST	TRICKS-XV	TRACS (4D-TRAK)	Freeze Frame 3D-DRKS
Non-contrast angiography	NATIVE	Flow Prepped Fiesta	TRANCE	FBI/CIA
High Resolution Bilateral Breast Imaging	VIEWS	VIBRANT-XV	BLISS	RADIANCE
Inversion Recovery	IR, Turbo IR	IR, MPIR. Fast IR	IR-TSE	IR
Short Tau IR	STIR	STIR	STIR	STIR
Long TAU IR	Turbo Dark Fluid	FLAIR	FLAIR	FLAIR
Turbo Spin Echo/Fast spin Echo	TSE	FSE	TSE	FSE
Single-Shot TSE/FSE	HASTE	SSFSE	SSTSE	FASE
T1 3D with fat suppression	VIBE	LAVA	THRIVE	QUICK 3D
T2 3D	Space	CUBE	VISTA	
FSE/TSE with 90 °Flip-Back Pulse	RESTORE	FRFSE	DRIVE	T2 Pulse FSE
Number of Echos	Turbo Factor	ETL, Echo Train Length	Turbo Factor	ETL
Time Between Echos	Echo Spacing	Echo Spacing	Echo Spacing	Echo Spacing
Echo Planar Imaging (EPI)	EPI	EPI	EPI	EPI
Diffusion Weighted Imaging	DWI	DWI	DWI	DWI

	Siemens	GE	Phillips	Toshiba
Motion Correction				
Motion Correction with Radial Blades	BLADE	PROPELLER	MultiVane	JET
Parallel Acquisition Techniques				
PAT: Image-based Algorithm	SENSE, GRAPPA	ASSET	SENSE	SPEEDER
Calibration Scan	Turbo-Calibration	Calibration for ASSET	CLEAR	Calibration for SPEEDER
Spectroscopy				
Prostate Spectroscopy	3D CSI	PROSE		
Breast Spectroscopy	GRACE	BREASE		
Sequence Parameters				
Repetition Time, Echo Time (in msec)	TR, TE	TR, TE	TR, TE	TR, TE
Inversion Time	TI	TI	TI	TI
Averages	Average	NEX	NSA	NAQ
RF Pulse in Gradient Echo	Flip Angle	Flip Angle	Flip Angle	Flip Angle
Scan Measurement Time	Acquisition Time, TA	Acquisition Time	Acquisition Time	Acquisition Time
Distance Between Slices	Distance Factor	GAP	GAP	GAP
Shifting Slices off Center	Off Center Shift	Off Center FOV	Off Center FOV	Phase &Frequency Shift
Field of View (FOV)	FOV [mm]	FOV [cm]	FOV [mm]	FOV [cm]

(Continued)

	Siemens	GE	Phillips	Toshiba
Rectangular FOV	FOV Phase	Rectangular FOV	Rectangular FOV	Rectangular FOV
Bandwidth	Bandwidth	Receive Bandwidth	Fat/ Water Shift	Bandwidth
Variable Bandwidth	Optimized Bandwidth	Variable Bandwidth	Optimized Bandwidth	Matched Bandwidth
Frequency Oversampling	Oversampling	Anti-Aliasing	Frequency Oversampling	Frequency Wrap Suppression
Phase oversampling	Phase Oversampling	No Phase Wrap	Fold-over S uppression	Phase Wrap Suppression
Segmented k-space	Lines/ Segments	Views per segment	Views/Segments	Segments
Half Fourier Imaging	Half Fourier	½ NEX	Half Scan	AFI
Gradient Moment Nulling	GMR/ Flow comp	Flow Comp	Flow Comp/ Flag	FC
Ramped FR Pulse	TONE	Ramped RF	TONE	ISCE
Magnetization Transfer Contrast	MTC/ MTS	MTC	MTC	SORS-STC
Fat Saturation-Chemically	Fat Sat	Fat Sat/ Chem Sat	SPIR	MSOFT
Water Excitation	Water Excitation	SPECIAL	Proset	PASTA
Fat/Water Separation (Dixon)	Dixon	IDEAL	Dixon	Dixon
Contrast Kinetics/ Time Resolved	Treat/ Twist	TRICKS	4D TRAK	3D DRKS
Prep Pulse-Spatially	Presat	SAT	REST	Pre Sat

	Siemens	GE	Phillips	Toshiba
Moving Sat Pulse	Travel Sat	Walking Sat	Travel REST	BFAST
Multi-channel RF coil sensitivity	Pre-scan normalization	PRUE	Clear	Leave Blank
Scan Synchronization with ECG	ECG triggered	Cardiac Gated	ECG Triggered/ VCG	Cardiac Gated
Delay after R-wave	Trigger Delay; TD	Trigger Delay; TD	Trigger Delay; TD	Trigger Delay; TD
Respiratory Gating	Respiratory Gated	Respiratory Gated	Trigger; PEAR	Respiratory Gated
Contrast Bolus Timing	CARE bolus	Fluoro Trigger	Bolus Trak	Visual Prep

Glossary of MRI Terms

A

Acceleration factor The multiplicative term by which faster imaging pulse sequences such as *multiple echo imaging* reduce total imaging time compared with conventional imaging sequences such as *spin echo imaging*.

Acoustic noise Vibrations of the gradient coil create sound waves. These vibrations are caused by interactions of the magnetic field created by pulses of the current through the gradient coil with the main magnetic field in a manner similar to a loudspeaker coil.

Acquisition matrix The number of sampling data in the phase-encoding and frequency-encoding directions.

Acquisition time The acquisition time is the time required to collect imaging data.

Active shimming Shimming is the process of making the magnetic field more uniform by suitably adjusting the currents in shim coils.

Aliasing Aliasing occurs when the area of anatomy extends beyond the field of view.

Analog to digital converter (ADC) Converts the received (analog) signals into digital data for compatibility with computer systems.

Angiography (MRA) An application to produce images of blood vessels. A common approach is to saturate stationary spins while increasing signal from the flowing blood.

Array coil RF coil composed of multiple separate elements that can be used individually or simultaneously.

Array processor A dedicated computer system specially designed to perform Fourier transformation and speed up numerical calculations needed for MR imaging.

Artifacts False information in the image produced by the imaging process or electrical or metal interference.

ASSET (Array Spatial Sensitivity Encoding Technique) A parallel imaging technique that uses multiple receiver coils to simultaneously collect different portions of the image in physical space, or different data points in k-space, which are then used to reconstruct collected images. Parallel imaging speeds data collection and therefore decreases total imaging time, with some loss in signal-to-noise ratios compared with conventional imaging. Also called SENSE, SMASH, GRAPPA, and iPAT.

Axial plane (transverse plane) The plane perpendicular to the long axis of the human body (head-to-foot).

B

Bo A conventional symbol for the constant magnetic (induction) field in an MR system.

B1 A conventional symbol for the radiofrequency magnetic induction field used in a MR system, usually transverse to Bo.

BOLD (Blood Oxygen Level Dependent) A fMRI technique to map areas of the brain that are responsible for a particular task. It measures the hemodynamic response (change in blood flow) related to neural activity. The patient performs a task, i.e., finger tapping, and the sensory motor cortex of the brain will respond by showing increased signal. Other mapping includes visual and auditory stimulation and memory tasks.

Balanced steady-state free precession An MR gradient echo pulse sequence designed to produce contrast weighted by the T2/T1 ratio, with higher SNR and reduced artifacts compared with SSFP. Specific vendor names for this sequence include True-Flash imaging with steady-state precession (True-FISP), fast imaging employing steady-state acquisition (FIESTA), and balanced fast-field echo (balanced-FFE).

Bandwidth A general term referring to a range of frequencies.

Bolus tracking A method of tracking contrast in the blood as it moves into the imaging plane.

BRAVO (BRAinVOlume) A 3-D high-resolution IR-Prepared FSPGR T1-weighted sequence. This technique provides whole-brain isotropic volumes.

BREASE A breast-specific spectroscopy application designed to increase diagnostic ability.

C

CBF Cerebral blood flow. The flow of capillary blood through the cortex, measured in units of flow (milliliters per minute) per unit mass of cortex.

CBV Cerebral blood volume. The volume of blood in a given volume of cerebral cortex, measured in units of volume.

Cardiac gating Acquisition of images synchronized with the cardiac cycle. A variety of means for detecting these cycles can be used, such as the ECG and peripheral pulse gating.

Chemical shift (d) A variation in the resonance frequency of a nuclear spin caused by the chemical environment around the nucleus.

Cine acquisition A collection of rapidly recorded sequential images displayed in a movie format.

Coil Single or multiple loops of wire designed to produce a magnetic field from current flowing through the wire, or to detect a changing magnetic field by voltage induced in the wire.

Contrast The difference in signal intensity of two adjacent regions of an image.

Contrast agent Substance administered to subject being imaged to alter selectively the image intensity of a particular anatomical or functional region, typically by reducing the relaxation times, including T1, T2, and T2*.

Coronal plane The imaging plane defined by the head-to-foot and left-to-right directions in the body. A stack of images acquired in the coronal plane separates images by their anterior-to-posterior locations.

Cosmic (Coherent Oscillatory State acquisition for the Manipulation of Imaging Contrast) A 3-D segmented multishot centric k-space technique that improves the CNR and SNR of cervical spine tissue, including the spinal cord, vertebral disks, nerve root canal, and contrast between cerebral spinal fluid and nerve.

Cryogen Very-low-temperature liquefied gas (helium or nitrogen) used to maintain superconducting magnets in a superconducting state.

CUBE Cube is a 3-D isotropic imaging technique with sub-millimeter spatial resolution and excellent contrast to help visualize even diminutive lesions. 3-D data from a single scan can be quickly and easily reconstructed into any plane with the same high resolution of the primary plane.

D

Dephasing The loss of magnetization in the transverse plane, typically because different magnetic dipoles of different nuclei are precessing about the main magnetic field, Bo, at slightly different precessional frequencies and therefore lose phase coherence.

Dephasing gradient Magnetic field gradient pulse used to create spatial variation of phase of transverse magnetization.

Diamagnetic A substance that will slightly decrease a magnetic field when placed within it (its magnetization is oppositely directed to the magnetic field, i.e., with a small negative magnetic susceptibility).

DTI (Diffusion Tensor Imaging) Tensor imaging and tractography are diffusion-based MR techniques for advanced functional imaging of brain white matter (WM). Imaging brain anisotropy can yield useful information about WM integrity and demonstrate pathology occult to conventional imaging techniques. It can also provide ordered WM tracts such as directional orientation and connectivity, which can be useful in the understanding of WM disease states.

DWI Diffusion-weighted imaging. DWI is an imaging technique that looks at the diffusion of water molecules by using field gradients. Restricted water molecules reflect areas of lower diffusion in demyelinization and cytotoxic edema. Areas of cerebral infarction have decreased apparent diffusion, which results in increased signal intensity "bright" on diffusion-weighted MRI scans. DWI has been demonstrated to be more sensitive for the early detection of stroke than standard pulse sequences and is closely related to temperature mapping.

Dipole Magnetic dipole. North and south magnetic poles separated by a finite distance.

E

Echo planar imaging (EPI) A single-shot gradient echo or spin-echo imaging technique that collects complete 2-D image data.

Echo spacing The time gap between successive echo peaks in a fast spin-echo pulse sequence.

Echo time (TE) The time in milliseconds between the application of the 90-degree pulse and the peak of the echo signal.

Echo train length (ETL) The number 180 RF rephrasing pulses in a fast spin-echo pulse sequence.

Excitation Putting energy into the spin system; if a net transverse magnetization is produced, an MR signal can be observed.

F

Faraday shield (Faraday Cage) An electrically conductive screen or shield that reduces or eliminates interference between outside radio waves and those from the MRI unit.

Fat suppression MRI pulse sequence techniques in which the signal from hydrogen-containing lipids (mostly CH2) is reduced compared with the signal from water-containing tissues.

Ferromagnetic A substance, such as iron, that has a large positive magnetic susceptibility.

Field of view (FOV) The rectangular region in physical space to which the MRI data collected corresponds. Its dimensions are independently controlled by the frequency-encode and phase-encode gradients.

FIESTA A 2-D and 3-D imaging technique that uses an ultrashort TR and TE steady-state acquisition sequence that provides images of fluid-filled structures with very short acquisition times. The FIESTA sequence uses the T2 steady-state contrast mechanism to provide high SNR images with strong signal from fluid tissues (i.e., blood) while suppressing background tissue for contrast and anatomic detail of small structures (IAC). Can be used for cardiac, IAC/trigeminal nerves, and vascular body imaging.

Flip angle Amount of rotation of the macroscopic magnetization vector produced by an RF pulse, with respect to the direction of the static magnetic field.

Flow compensation Means of reducing flow effects, e.g., gradient moment nulling.

Flow void The occurrence of low signal in regions of blood flow.

Fourier transform (FT) A mathematical procedure to separate out the frequency components of a signal from its amplitudes as a function of time, or vice versa.

Free induction decay (FID) If transverse magnetization of the spins is produced, e.g., by a 90° pulse, a transient MR signal will result that will decay toward zero with a characteristic time constant T2 (or T2*); this decaying signal is the FID.

Frequency (f) The number of repetitions of a periodic process per unit of time. Cycles/seconds.

Frequency encoding The process of locating a MR signal in one dimension by applying a magnetic field gradient along that dimension during the period when the signal is being received.

Fringe field A term usually relating to the extent of the magnetic field surrounding the magnet.

Functional magnetic resonance imaging (fMRI) The use of MRI to study function in addition to anatomy. In the brain, fMRI measures changes in cerebral blood flow and cerebral blood oxygenation as correlates of neuronal activity.

G

G_x, G_y, G_z Conventional symbols for magnetic field gradient. Used with subscripts to denote spatial direction component of gradient, i.e., direction along which the field changes.

Gadolinium A paramagnetic MR contrast that strongly decreases the T1 relaxation times of the tissues to which it has access. Although toxic by itself, it can be given safely in a chelated form such as Gd-DTPA, which still retains much of its strong effect on relaxation times.

Gating *Synchronization* of imaging with a phase of the cardiac or respiratory cycles. A variety of means for detecting these cycles can be used, such as the ECG, peripheral pulse, chest motion, etc. The synchronization can be *prospective* or *retrospective*.

Gauss (G) A unit of magnetic field strength. 1 Tesla = 10,000 Gauss.

Gibbs phenomenon Artifactual ripples that occur near a discontinuity when reconstructing a mathematical function from only a finite portion of its *Fourier transform*. In MR imaging, it can be seen as linear artifacts parallel to sharp edges in the object, particularly with the use of *zero filling*.

Gradient coils Current carrying coils designed to produce a desired magnetic field gradient (so that the magnetic field will be stronger in some locations than others). Proper design of the size and configuration of the coils is necessary to produce a controlled and uniform gradient.

Gradient-echo A signal echo produced by reversing the direction of a magnetic field gradient or by applying balanced pulses of magnetic field gradient before and after a refocusing RF pulse.

Gradient-echo pulse sequence A pulse sequence that relies on gradient reversal to rephase the transverse magnetization, using variable flip angles.

Gyromagnetic ratio The ratio of the magnetic moment to the angular momentum of a particle. This is a constant for a given nucleus.

H

Hemodynamic response Changes in blood flow, blood volume, and blood oxygenation as a result of local neural activity.

Hertz (Hz) The standard unit of frequency.

Homogeneity Uniformity.

I

IDEAL IDEAL uses a fat/water separation DIXON technique to consistent, robust fat and water separation every time, even in difficult-to-scan anatomies and in the presence of metal implants. Four different contrasts: water only, fat only, in-phase, and out-of-phase are generated from a single acquisition, for confident diagnoses and fewer repeats. The "water only" image achieves superior fat sat, whereas a "fat only" visualizes fatty lesions. IDEAL provides unique fat suppression capabilities on the hips, shoulders, and spine.

Isotropic imaging Imaging in which voxel dimensions are equal in x, y, and z directions.

Inductance Measure of the magnetic coupling between two current-carrying loops (mutual) reflecting their spatial relationship or of a loop (such as a coil) with itself (self). One of the principal determinants of the resonance frequency of an RF circuit.

Induction (B) See *Magnetic induction*.

Inhomogeneity Degree of lack of homogeneity, for example, the fractional deviation of the local magnetic field from the average value of the field.

In-phase image An image in which the signals from two spectral components (such as fat and water) add constructively in a voxel.

Interleaved image acquisition The joint collection of data for two or more separate images such that a subset of k-space samples for the second image is acquired immediately after that for the first image. This method avoids misregistration between the two images and allows for accurate subtraction of the two images.

Inversion-recovery (IR) Pulsed MR imaging sequence wherein the nuclear magnetization is inverted at a time on the order of T1 before the regular imaging pulse-gradient sequences. A 180° inversion pulse is applied and an interval TI (inversion time) is weighted and then a 90° pulse is applied, after which the MR signal is measured. The TI interval is used to let the longitudinal magnetization recover through spin-lattice or T1 relaxation. After the initial TI, a 90° pulse is used to rotate the available longitudinal magnetization onto the transverse plane to generate a signal. Tissues with fast T1 recovery will have a larger longitudinal magnetization at the end of TI, thus will produce a stronger signal after the 90° pulse. Therefore, in T1-weighted images, bright tissue represents short T1 and dark tissue long T1.

Inversion time See *TI*.

Isocenter, magnetic The position in the magnet that is centered in the x, y, and z directions. At this location, the static magnetic field is typically highest in uniformity.

Isotropic voxel A voxel with equal physical dimensions in x, y, and z directions.

K

Kilohertz (kHz) Unit of frequency; equal to 1000 hertz.

k-space Mathematical space in which the Fourier transform of the image is represented. The data acquired for MR image reconstruction generally correspond to samples of k-space, that is, they represent values of the Fourier transform of the image at a particular set of locations in k-space. See also *Spatial frequency*.

k-space filling The location and order of obtaining data in two-dimensional spatial frequency space (k-space). For example, conventional MR pulse sequences such as spin-echo and gradient-echo imaging fill a single line of k-space with each data measurement. A different phase-encoding step is used to fill out another parallel line of k-space. The full set of measurements completes a Cartesian grid of points in k-space. Other options for k-space filling include radial filling (back-projection imaging) or spiral filling (spiral imaging).

L

Larmor frequency (fo) Frequency = Gyromagnetic ratio of an element (Hydrogen) × the Field Strength of the Magnet. Gyromagnetic ratio of Hydrogen is = 42.576 Mhz at 1 Tesla

Lattice In MR, the magnetic and thermal environment with which nuclei exchange energy in T1 longitudinal relaxation.

LAVA (Liver Acquisition with Volume Acceleration) A 3-D FastSPGR technique that combines contrast-enhanced, multiphasic imaging with superb fat suppression for imaging of the abdomen with high resolution and large coverage in one breath-hold. LAVA acquires a stack of overlapping thin slices with high in-plane resolution that produces images of the arterial, portal, and venous phases. There is exceptional contrast differentiates between the liver and spleen, revealing the subtle details you need to make the best diagnosis. This not only precisely depicts anatomy and contrast uptake, but also contains vascular information that can be easily revealed by postprocessing.

Line width Spread in frequency of a resonance line in a MR spectrum.

Longitudinal magnetization (Mz) Component of the Mz of the net magnetization vector along the static magnetic field. After excitation by RF pulse, the vector returns to equilibrium value at a rate characteristic of time constant T1.

Longitudinal relaxation Return of longitudinal magnetization to its equilibrium value after excitation; requires exchange of energy between the nuclear spins and the lattice.

Longitudinal relaxation time Time constant T1, which determines rate of equilibrium within the lattice.

M

M Conventional symbol for magnetization vector.

Mxy Transverse magnetization.

Mz Longitudinal magnetization.

Mo Equilibrium value of the magnetization; directed along the direction of the static magnetic field, Bo.

Magnetic dipole North and south magnetic poles separated by a finite distance. An electric current loop can create an equivalent magnetic dipole.

Magnetic field (H) The region surrounding the magnet processing its conductive properties. Magnetic field is a vector quantity, which is the direction of the field and produces a magnetizing force on a body within it.

Magnetic field gradient A magnetic field that changes in strength in a certain given direction. Such fields are used in MR imaging with selective excitation to select a region for imaging and also to encode the location of MR signals received from the object being imaged. Measured (e.g.) in teslas per meter.

Magnetic fringe field The region surrounding a magnet and exhibiting a magnetic field strength that is significantly higher than the earth's magnetic field. Because of the physical properties of magnetic fields, the magnetic flux that penetrates the useful volume of the magnet will return through the surroundings of the magnet to form closed field lines.

Magnetic induction (B) Also called *magnetic flux density*. The net magnetic effect from an externally applied magnetic field and the resulting magnetization.

Magnetic moment A measure of the net magnetic properties of an object or particle. A nucleus with an intrinsic spin will have an associated magnetic dipole moment, so that it will interact with a magnetic field (as if it were a tiny bar magnet).

Magnetic resonance (MR) The absorption or emission of electromagnetic energy by nuclei or electrons in a static magnetic field, after RF excitation pulses are applied. The resonance frequency is proportional to the magnetic field, and is given by the Larmor equation. Only unpaired electrons or nuclei exhibit magnetic resonance.

Magnetic resonance angiography (MRA) Angiography using MRI.

Magnetic resonance imaging (MRI) Imaging the distribution of mobile hydrogen nuclei (protons) in the body. The image brightness depends jointly on the spin density (PD) and the relaxation times (T1 and T2).

Magnetic resonance spectroscopy (MRS) Use of magnetic resonance to study the MR spectrum of a sample of a tissue. Because nuclei of different elements resonate at different frequencies, elements in the sample contribute a different frequency component. A chemical analysis is done to analyze the MR signal response.

Magnetic shielding The means of confining the strong magnetic field surrounding the magnet. Most commonly the use of material with high permeability (passive shielding) or by using secondary counteracting coils outside of the primary coils (active shielding).

Magnetic susceptibility The extent to which a material becomes magnetized when placed in a magnetic field.

Magnetization transfer contrast (MTC) A technique that selectively alters tissue contrast on the basis of micromolecular environment. It produces change in relative signal intensities by applying an off-resonance pulse to the water peak. It is applied at +1000 Hz, opposite side of fat saturation pulse at −220 Hz. This improves contrast by saturating the short T2 components of tissue such as gray/white matter and skeletal muscle. MTC is often used in MRA to suppress background tissue while preserving signal intensity from blood vessels, resulting in increased vessel visualization

Magnetization vector The summation of all the individual nuclear magnetic moments with positive magnetization value at equilibrium vs. those in a random state.

Matrix size The number of data points collected in one, two, or all three directions. Normally used for the 2-D in-plane sampling. The display matrix may be different from the acquisition matrix, although resolution is determined by the latter.

Maximum intensity projection (MIP) A technique for producing multiple projection images from a volume of image data (i.e., 3-D volume or a stack of 2-D slices). The volume of image data is processed along a selected angle and the pixel with the highest signal intensity is projected onto a 2-D image.

Megahertz (MHz) Unit of frequency, equal to one million hertz.

MERGE (Multi-Echo Recalled Gradient Echo) A 2-D and 3-D T2* gradient echo where signals from several different TEs are averaged and those echoes form a single T2*-weighted image. It uses a large receiver bandwidth that reduces chemical and susceptibly artifacts, which improves image tissue contrast. The sequence also provides better fat suppression and brighter signal intensity from fluid than conventional GRE sequence.

MRA See *Magnetic resonance angiography*.

MRI See *Magnetic resonance imaging*.

MRS See *Magnetic resonance spectroscopy*.

MTC See *Magnetization transfer contrast*.

Multiple echo imaging Spin-echo imaging or echo-train pulse sequence techniques such fast spin-echo (FSE), rapid acquisition with relaxation enhancement (RARE), or turbo spin-echo (TSE) techniques in which more than one 180-degree echo is acquired per TR echo-train or RARE techniques speed image acquisition by filling multiple lines of k-space per TR.

Multiple slice imaging Variation of sequential plane imaging techniques that can be used with selective excitation techniques that do not affect adjacent slices. Adjacent slices are imaged while waiting for relaxation of the first slice toward equilibrium, resulting in decreased image acquisition time for the set of slices.

N

NEX See *NSA*.

NMR imaging Creation of images of the body by use of the nuclear magnetic resonance phenomenon.

Noise That component of the reconstructed image caused by random and unpredictable processes as opposed to the signal within the image itself, which is a result of predictable processes not to be confused with artifacts, which are nonrandom errors in the image.

NSA Number of signals averaged together to determine each distinct position-encoded signal to be used in image reconstruction.

Nuclear spin An intrinsic property of certain nuclei that gives them an associated characteristic angular momentum and magnetic moment.

O

Off resonance A state occurring when the Larmor frequency of a spin is different from that of the exciting RF field.

On resonance A state occurring when the Larmor frequency of a spin is the same as that of the exciting RF field.

Opposed-phase image An image in which the signal from two spectral components (such as fat and water) are 180° out-of-phase and lead to destructive interference in a voxel.

P

Parallel imaging The use of multiple receiver coils to collect simultaneously different portions of the image in physical space, or different data points in k-space, which are then used to reconstruct collected images. Parallel imaging speeds data collection and therefore decreases total imaging time. Particular strategies in parallel imaging include vendor-specific methods such as sensitivity-encoding (SENSE, mSENSE), simultaneous acquisition of spatial harmonics (SMASH), generalized auto-calibrating partially parallel acquisition (GRAPPA), integrated parallel acquisition techniques (iPAT), and others.

Paramagnetic A substance with a small but positive magnetic susceptibility that reduces the relaxation times of hydrogen. Typical paramagnetic substances usually possess an unpaired electron and include atoms or ions of transition elements, rare earth elements, some metals, and some molecules including molecular oxygen and free radicals.

Partial Fourier imaging Reconstruction of an image from an MR dataset comprising an asymmetric sampling of *k-space*. For example, it can be used either to shorten *image acquisition time* by reducing the number of *phase encoding* steps required, or shorten the *echo time, TE,* by moving the *echo* off center in the *acquisition window*. In either case, the *signal-to-noise ratio* is reduced and the resolution can be improved to correspond to the maximum available resolution in the data.

Partial volume effect The loss of contrast between two adjacent tissues in an image caused by insufficient *resolution* so that more than one tissue type occupies the same *voxel* (or *pixel*).

Passive shielding *Magnetic shielding* through the use of high *permeability* material (see also *Magnetic shielding, Self-shielding,* and *Room shielding*).

Passive shimming *Shimming* by adjusting the position of suitable pieces of *ferromagnetic* metal within or around the main magnet of an *MR* system.

Phase In a periodic function (such as rotational or sinusoidal motion), the position relative to a particular part of the cycle.

Perfusion-weighted imaging (PWI) A technique that provides metabolic and hemodynamic data of the brain based on the negative enhancement of the brain when injecting contrast rapidly and viewed over time.

Phase encoding Encoding the distribution of sources of *MR signals* along a direction in space with different phases by applying a pulsed *magnetic field gradient* along that direction before detection of the signal. In general, it is necessary to acquire a set of signals with a suitable set of different phase-encoding gradient pulses to reconstruct the distribution of the sources along the encoded direction.

Pixel Acronym for a picture element; the smallest discrete part of a digital image display.

Planar imaging Imaging technique in which the image of a plane is built up from signals received from the whole plane.

PROPELLER (Periodically Rotated Overlapping ParallEL Lines with Enhanced Reconstruction) A technique that significantly reduces the effects of motion artifacts by filling k-space in a blade manner oversampling center and throwing out the bad data during reconstruction of the image. PROPELLER reduces motion artifacts without compromising image resolution or prolonging scan time. Presently, PROPELLER can be acquired with routine T2, T2 FLAIR, and DWI scanning of the brain. PROPELLER also reduces artifacts caused by magnetic susceptibility and optimizes signal and noise contrast, helping to visualize even small or subtle lesions.

Proton density (PD) The quantity of hydrogen nuclei in each voxel or volume of tissue. Spin-echo imaging can generate a proton density-weighted image by using long TR and very short TE settings.

PRUE A coil signal intensity correction that uses a coil intensity profile calibration to better equalize signal intensity from multi-channel coils. A calibration scan is required before applying PRUE to the acquisition.

Pulse, 90° (π/2 pulse) *RF pulse* designed to rotate the *macroscopic magnetization vector* 90° in space as referred to the *rotating frame of reference*, usually about an axis at right angles to the main *magnetic field*. If the spins are initially aligned with the magnetic field, this pulse will produce *transverse magnetization* and an *FID*.

Pulse, 180° (π pulse) *RF pulse* designed to rotate the *macroscopic magnetization vector* 180° in space as referred to the *rotating frame of reference*, usually about an axis at right angles to the main *magnetic field*. If the *spins* are initially aligned with the magnetic field, this pulse will produce *inversion*.

Pulse sequences Set of *RF* (and/or *gradient*) *magnetic field pulses* and time spacings between these pulses; used in conjunction with magnetic field gradients and MR signal reception to produce *MR images*. Varying parameters that generate a particular image is to list the repetition time (*TR*), the echo time (*TE*), and, if using inversion-recovery, the inversion time, TI, with all times given in milliseconds. For example, 2500/30/1000 would indicate an inversion-recovery pulse sequence with TR of 2500 msec, TE of 30 msec, and TI of 1000 msec.

Q

Quadrature coil A *coil* that produces an *RF* field with circular polarization by providing RF feed points that are out of *phase* by 90°.

Quenching Loss of *superconductivity* of the current-carrying *coil* that may occur unexpectedly in a superconducting magnet. As the magnet becomes resistive, heat will be released, which can result in rapid evaporation of liquid helium in the *cryostat*. This may present a hazard if not properly planned for.

R

Radiofrequency (RF) The wave *frequency* that is intermediate between auditory and infrared. The RF used in *MR* studies is commonly in the *megahertz* (MHz) range. The principal effect of RF *magnetic fields* on the body is power deposition in the form of heating, mainly at the surface; this is a principal area of concern for safety limits.

Receiver coil Coil of the *RF receiver*; "picks up" the *MR signal*.

Region-of-interest (ROI) A user-defined subset of pixels in a planar image.

Relaxation The return of an excited system of spinning magnetic dipoles (spins) to its equilibrium state.

Relaxation rates Reciprocals of the *relaxation times*, $T1$ and $T2$ ($R1 = 1/T1$ and $R2 = 1/T2$). There is often a linear relation between the concentration of MR *contrast agents* and the resulting change in relaxation rate.

Relaxation times After *excitation*, the *spins* will tend to return to their equilibrium distribution, in which there is no *transverse magnetization* and the *longitudinal magnetization* is at its maximum value and oriented in the direction of the static *magnetic field*. It is observed that in the absence of applied *RF magnetic field*, the transverse magnetization decays toward zero with a characteristic time constant $T2$, and the longitudinal magnetization returns toward the equilibrium value Mo with a characteristic time constant $T1$.

Repetition time See *TR*.

Rephasing gradient *Magnetic field gradient pulse* applied to reverse the spatial variation of *phase of transverse magnetization* caused by a *dephasing gradient*. For example, in *selective excitation*, it is a magnetic field gradient applied for a brief period after a selective excitation pulse, in the opposite direction to the gradient used for the selective excitation. The result of the gradient reversal is a rephasing of the *spins* (which will have gotten out of phase with each other along the direction of the selection gradient), forming a *gradient echo* and improving the sensitivity of imaging after the selective excitation process.

Resonance A large-amplitude vibration in a mechanical or electrical system caused by a relatively small periodic stimulus with a *frequency* at or close to a natural frequency of the system; in *MR* apparatus, resonance can refer to the NMR itself or to the tuning of the *RF* circuitry.

Resonance frequency *Frequency* at which *resonance* phenomenon occurs; given by the *Larmor equation*.

RF See *Radiofrequency*.

RF coil *Coil* used for transmitting *RF pulses* and/or receiving *MR signals*.

RF pulse Burst of *RF magnetic field* delivered to object by *RF transmitter*. For *RF frequency* near the *Larmor frequency*, it will result in rotation of the *macroscopic magnetization vector* in the *rotating frame of reference*. The amount of rotation will depend on the strength and duration of the RF pulse; commonly used examples are 90° ($\pi/2$) and 180° (π) *pulses*.

RF shielding Electrically conducting shielding designed to isolate an MR system from its environment at the *resonant frequencies* of interest.

RF spoiling The use of varying *phase* or timing of the *RF pulses* to prevent setting up a condition of *steady-state free precession*, e.g., in *rapid-excitation MR imaging*.

Room shielding *Magnetic shielding* through the use of high *permeability* material in the walls (plus floor and ceiling) of the magnet room. Room shielding can be complete (e.g., six sides of a box), or partial if the *fringe field* is to be reduced only in certain areas (see also *Magnetic shielding*).

S

Safety Safety concerns in MR include *magnetic field* strength, *RF* heating *(SAR)*–induced currents caused by rapidly varying magnetic fields *(dB/dt)*, effects on implanted devices such as *pacemakers*, magnetic *torque* effects on indwelling metal such as clips and possible "missile effect" of *magnetic forces*, and *acoustic noise*.

Sagittal plane The plane defined by the head-to-foot and anterior-to-posterior directions in the human body. A stack of images acquired in the sagittal plane separates images by their left-to-right locations. The midline sagittal plane bisects the left and right half of the human body.

SAR See *Specific absorption rate*.

Saturation A nonequilibrium state in MR in which equal numbers of spins are aligned against and with the magnetic field, so that there is no net magnetization. Can be produced by repeatedly applying RF pulses at the Larmor frequency with interpulse times short compared with T1, producing incomplete realignment of the net magnetization with the static magnetic field.

Saturation pulses Sequence of *RF* (and *gradient*) pulses designed to produce saturation, typically in a selected region or set of regions, most often by the use of *selective excitation* followed by a *spoiler pulse*. Can be used to reduce signal from flowing blood by saturating regions upstream from the region being imaged.

SCIC (Surface Coil Intensity Correction) This function equalizes the signal *intensity* when multichannel coils are used. The signal *intensity* of the region close to the *coil* is reduced and produces a more homogenous image.

Shim coils *Coils* carrying a relatively small current that are used to provide auxiliary *magnetic fields* to compensate for *inhomogeneity* in the main magnetic field of an *MR* system.

Shimming Correction of *inhomogeneity* of the *magnetic field* produced by the main magnet of an *MR* system because of imperfections in the magnet or from the presence of external *ferromagnetic* objects.

Signal averaging The averaging together of signals acquired under the same or similar conditions so as to suppress the effects of random variations or random artifacts. The number of signals averaged together can be abbreviated to *NSA*.

Signal-to-noise ratio (SNR or S/N) Used to describe the relative contributions to a detected signal of the true signal and random superimposed signals (*"noise"*) (NSA). One common method to improve (increase) the SNR is to average several measurements of the signal. Can be improved by sampling larger volumes (with a corresponding loss of spatial resolution) or, within limits, by increasing the strength of the magnetic field used. *Surface coils* can also be used to improve local SNR. The SNR will depend, in part, on the electrical properties of the sample or patient being studied.

Signal suppression The elimination or reduction of a particular signal by, for example, the application of a narrow-band *frequency*-selective preparation pulse centered at the *resonant* frequency of the signal. This can also be accomplished using an *inversion recovery* technique to null the signal as it recovers its longitudinal magnetization.

Single-shot imaging The process of acquiring all data needed to form a 2-D image with a single excitation pulse. *Echo-planar imaging* is an example of single-shot imaging

Slice The effective physical extent of the "planar" region being imaged.

Slice selection The excitation of spins in a limited planar section of tissue by applying a gradient (the slice-selective gradient) while sending a narrow-band RF pulse of appropriate frequencies into the subject.

Slice thickness The thickness of a slice is the distance between the points. It is a 2-D or 3-D volume of imaged area that affects SNR, spatial resolution, and partial volume effects.

S/N and SNR See *Signal-to-noise ratio*.

Spatial frequency A dimension of the *Fourier transform* space (*k-space* representation of an image), having units of inverse distance. Higher values of spatial frequencies correspond to finer detail in the image.

Spatial resolution The smallest distance between two points in the object that can be distinguished as separate details in the image, generally indicated as a length or a number of black and white line pairs per millimeter.

SPECIAL A uniform fat suppression technique that improves the image quality on high-definition 3-D imaging.

Specific absorption rate (SAR [W/kg]) Time varying electromagnetic fields can deposit energy in tissues. This energy is deposited mostly in the form of heat, which is considered the primary mechanism of biological effect. The SAR is defined as the energy dissipated in tissue (watts) per kilogram of tissue mass.

Spectroscopic imaging MR techniques that permit acquisition of an MR spectrum for each pixel or voxel in the MR image. The resulting acquired data can then be presented as an MR spectrum for each pixel or voxel, or as an image or set of images that reflect(s) the intensity of a particular spectral peak at each spatial location in two or three dimensions. The methods may be used to sample a single region in space (single-voxel method) or multiple regions simultaneously (multi-voxel methods)

Spin The intrinsic *angular momentum* of an elementary particle, or system of particles such as a nucleus, that is also responsible for the *magnetic moment*; or, a particle or nucleus possessing such a spin. The spins of nuclei have characteristic fixed values. Pairs of neutrons and protons align to cancel out their spins so that nuclei with an odd number of neutrons and/or protons will have a net nonzero rotational component.

Spin echo (SE) The *RF pulse sequence* whereby a 90° excitation pulse is followed by a 180° refocusing pulse.

Spin-lattice relaxation time See *T1*.

Spin-spin relaxation time See *T2*.

Spoiler gradient pulse Magnetic field *gradient* pulse applied to effectively remove *transverse magnetization* by producing a rapid variation of its *phase* along the direction of the gradient.

Steady-state coherent A state of *spins* that leads to an equilibrium *magnetization* for the longitudinal and transverse magnetization, or, when the magnetization at or after each *RF* pulse is the same as in the previous pulse.

Steady state free precession (SFP or SSFP) Method of *MR excitation* in which strings of *RF pulses* are applied rapidly and repeatedly with short interpulse intervals compared with both *T1* and *T2*. Alternating the *phases* of the RF pulses by 180° can be useful. The MR signal reforms as an *echo* immediately before each RF pulse; immediately after the RF pulse, there is additional signal from the *FID* produced by the pulse. The strength of the FID will depend on the time between pulses *(TR)*, the magnetization of the tissue, and the *flip angle* of the pulse; the strength of the echo will additionally depend on the T2 of the tissue.

Susceptibility artifact The loss of MR signal in voxels or regions with varying magnetic susceptibility (magnetic nonuniformities) caused by greater T2* decay. Susceptibility artifacts are more obvious in pulse sequences weighted more heavily by T2* effects, such as gradient-echo imaging.

T-U

T See *Tesla*.

T_1 or T1 ("T-one") Spin-lattice or longitudinal *relaxation time*; the characteristic time constant for *spins* to tend to align themselves with the external *magnetic field*. The time required for the net magnetization to grow to 63% of its final amplitude.

T1-weighted (T1W) Often used to indicate an image where most of the contrast between tissues or tissue states is caused by differences in tissue *T1*. T1 contrast is acquired using a short TR and a *short TE*.

T2 or T2 ("T-two") Spin-spin or transverse *relaxation time*; the characteristic time constant for loss of *phase* coherence among spins oriented at an angle to the static *magnetic field*, caused by interactions between the spins, with resulting loss of *transverse magnetization* and *MR signal*. The time at which the transverse magnetization has decayed to 37% of its full value as a result entirely of spin-spin interaction.

T2* ("T-two-star") The observed time constant of the *FID* as a result of loss of *phase* coherence among spins oriented at an angle to the static *magnetic field*, commonly caused by a combination of magnetic field *inhomogeneity*.

T2-weighted (T2W) Often used to indicate an image where most of the contrast between tissues or tissue states is the result of differences in tissue *T2*. T2 contrast state is acquired using a *long TR* and *long TE*.

Tailored pulse Shaped pulse whose magnitude (and possibly phase) is varied with time in a predetermined manner. Affects the *frequency* components of an *RF pulse* in a manner determined by the *Fourier transform* of the pulse.

TE Echo time. Time between middle of exciting (e.g., 90°) *RF pulse* and middle of *spin-echo* production.

TE min The shortest possible TE time for a given prescription, used to minimize flow dephasing and T2 effects.

Temporal resolution The shortest time duration between two events that can be measured with an MR experiment.

Tesla (T) The preferred *(SI)* unit of magnetic flux density. One tesla is equal to 10,000 *gauss*.

TI Inversion time. In *inversion recovery*, time between middle of *inverting (180°) RF pulse* and middle of the subsequent *exciting (90°)* pulse to detect amount of *longitudinal magnetization*.

Time-of-flight A 2-D or 3-D imaging technique that relies primarily on flow-related enhancement to distinguish moving spins from stationary spins. Blood that has flowed into the slice will not have experienced RF pulse saturation and will therefore appear brighter than stationary tissue.

Torque A *vector* quantity given by the vector product of the force and the position vector where the force is applied; for a rotating body, the torque is the product of the moment of inertia and the resulting angular acceleration.

TR Repetition time. The period of time between the beginning of a *pulse sequence* and the beginning of the succeeding (essentially identical) pulse sequence.

Transmit/receive (T/R) coil An *RF coil* that acts as both a transmitter (T) producing the *B1 excitation field*, and as a receiver (R) of the MR signal. Such a coil requires a T/R switching circuit to switch between the two modes. A body coil is typically a T/R coil, but smaller volume T/R coils (head/extremities) are often used at high field as a means of reducing RF power absorption.

Transverse magnetization (M_{xy}) Component of the *macroscopic magnetization vector* at right angles to the static *magnetic field (B0)*. *Precession* of the *transverse magnetization* at the *Larmor frequency* is responsible for the detectable *MR signal*. In the absence of externally applied *RF magnetic field*, the transverse magnetization will decay to zero with a characteristic time constant of *T2* or *T2**.

Transverse relaxation The loss of magnetization in the plane perpendicular to the static magnetic field, Bo.

Transverse relaxation time See *T2*.

Traveling saturation pulse A *saturation pulse* that moves from one spatial location to another for each *RF pulse* excitation or each MR slice acquired.

TRICKS (Time Resolved Imaging of Contrast KineticS) A 3-D dynamic contrast-enhanced imaging technique that captures flow dynamics of the vascular system over time. TRICKS MRA achieves high temporal resolution through k-space segment sharing. This addresses the trade-off between spatial and temporal resolution that is typical of conventional MR angiography. TRICKS can assess blood flow dynamics and visualize small caliber vessels.

Trigger In cardiac/respiratory gating, signal sent by the cardiac/respiratory monitor to activate data acquisition

Trigger delay time The time after *triggering* at which data acquisition takes place.

Trigger delay The time between the occurrence of the triggering pulse and the actual onset of imaging.

Trigger window (TW) In cardiac gating, a period during which no further data can be acquired. During this period, the system waits for the next R-wave trigger, which initiates a new sequence of data acquisition

Triggering Generation of an electrical pulse, upon detection of a physiological signal, which can be used to initiate a *synchronized* data acquisition *pulse sequence*.

Tuning Process of adjusting the *resonant frequency*, e.g., of the *RF circuit*, to the desired value, e.g., the *Larmor frequency*.

V

Variable flip angle The temporal variation of *flip angle* (from one *RF pulse* to the next) to enhance *SNR* and/or equalize the signal intensity for each *phase-encoding* step.

Variable TE The variation of *echo time* from one *RF pulse* to the next.

Variable TR The variation of *repetition time* from one *RF pulse* to the next.

Vector A quantity having both magnitude and direction, frequently represented by an arrow whose length is proportional to the magnitude and with an arrowhead at one end to indicate the direction.

Velocity encoding (VENC) A value entered to prescribe the highest velocities to be encoded without aliasing in phase contrast angiography

VIBRANT (Volume Imaging for BReast AssessmeNT) A FSPGR high-definition bilateral breast in both sagittal and axial planes in a single exam without trading off spatial or temporal resolution or compromising resolution or scan time. Eliminates fat with absolute reliability and confidence.

Volume of interest (VOI) A user-selected subset of voxels in a 3-D dataset.

Volume imaging Imaging techniques in which *MR signals* are gathered from the whole object volume to be imaged at once, with appropriate encoding *pulse RF and gradient sequences* to encode positions of the *spins*. Advantages include potential improvement in *signal-to-noise ratio* by including signal from the whole volume at once; disadvantages include a bigger computational task for image reconstruction and longer *image acquisition times* (although the entire volume can be imaged from the one set of data). Also called *simultaneous volume imaging* or *three-dimensional Fourier transform (3DFT) imaging*.

Voxel Volume element; the element of 3-D space corresponding to a pixel, for a given slice thickness.

W

Water-suppression The elimination or reduction of water signal from the image by application of a narrow-band frequency-selective pulse centered around the *resonant frequency* of the tissue.

X

x Dimension at right angles to the direction of the static *magnetic field (Bo or Ho)*, *z*, and orthogonal to *y*, the other dimension in this plane. This is commonly defined to be in the direction of the *frequency-encoding gradient*.

Y

y Dimension orthogonal to the direction of the static *magnetic field (Bo and Ho)*, *z*, and orthogonal to *x*, the other dimension in this plane. This is commonly defined to be in the direction of the *phase-encoding gradient*.

Z

z Dimension in the direction of the static *magnetic field (Bo and Ho)*, in both the stationary and *rotating frames of reference*. This is commonly defined to be in the direction of the *slice selection gradient*.

Zero filling Substitution of zeroes for unmeasured data points to increase the matrix size of the new data before *Fourier transformation* of *MR data*. This can be equivalent to performing an interpolation in the transformed data, resulting in *pixels* smaller than the actual *resolution* of the image.

Index

Note: Page numbers followed by "b" indicate boxes; "f" figures; "t" tables.

INDEX

INDEX